This is
COCAINE

Printed and bound in the UK by MPG Books, Bodmin

Published by Sanctuary Publishing Limited, Sanctuary House,
45-53 Sinclair Road, London W14 ONS, United Kingdom

www.sanctuarypublishing.com

Copyright: Sanctuary Publishing Limited, 2002

ISBN: 1-86074-423-0

This is
COCAINE

NICK CONSTABLE

CONTENTS

	INTRODUCTION	7
01	**CULTURE**	13
02	**WORLD**	45
03	**HISTORY**	75
04	**HEALTH**	115
05	**MONEY**	149
	ADDITIONAL INFO	177
	INDEX	187

INTRODUCTION

> **Charlie** *slang*
> 1 A fool *(Brit)*
> 2 *(in pl)* A woman's breasts *(Brit)*
> 3 Street term for cocaine *(US/Brit)*

There's someone you've got to meet. His name's Charlie and he gets to go to all the best parties. He's the club king of London and New York, mixes with pop stars and celebrities, has loads of contacts on Wall Street and is just about everyone's best friend in TV land. When Charlie's around you feel like a million dollars and when he leaves it's such a let-down. He's totally cool. Just treat him with a little respect.

Respect is about right. Around the world cocaine is more accessible than ever, and yet the social and scientific arguments swirling around it seem to get denser by the year. Coke is not the kind of drug you place in a tidy little box because everything about it defies simple analysis. Suffice to say that it is a substance of contradiction, of euphoria and despair; of obscene wealth and dire poverty. It knows no social barriers. Use it wisely and you'll be fine. Or maybe not.

CHARLIE'S FRIENDS

We're talking about the champagne drug of celebrities, yet loads of addicts are beggars and prostitutes. Its chemistry sustains Peruvian hill farmers just as much as sharp-suited banking professionals. You can be an occasional snorter for years and not have a problem but get psychologically hooked with surprising speed if you smoke it. Some say the drug guarantees great sex, others just want to re-organize their mantelpiece. You'll sell a line to your best friend with a clear conscience yet you know, deep down, that you've joined an industry that maims and kills to protect its markets.

By the way, got any cocaine on you? Bet you have. It may be that the only white powder looming large in your life comes from the vending machine at your local launderette, but Charlie gets everywhere. Especially into your purse or wallet.

HE'S A POPULAR GUY

In 1999, a BBC survey conducted by the forensic chemists Mass Spec Analytical discovered that out of 500 banknotes circulating in London, 99 per cent carried traces of cocaine. About 1 in 20 produced a particularly high reading, suggesting they had been used to snort it. The rest had probably been contaminated during handling by users and dealers.

Joe Reevy of Mass Spec explained (*Guardian*, 4 October 1999), 'Once you've taken a snort, the compounds will be in the oils of your skin and they'll get transferred to the notes you handle. That's the main way in which the cocaine gets on to the notes. When you test notes that have been used directly to snort cocaine you get a great big reading and the machine takes quite a while to settle down. You don't miss the difference.'

This study came less than a month after the government-backed British crime survey concluded that cocaine was the fastest-growing recreational drug among 20 to 24 year olds. Two years later, in April 2001, *The Face* magazine published a survey of 1,000 16 to 24 year olds, which showed that more than half of those questioned had taken it. *Face* editor Johnny Davis said prices as low as £10 ($14) per gram (that really is bargain-basement stuff) had attracted this new custom.

'Our suspicion, borne out by the findings, is that cocaine users are younger and more varied than ever before,' he said. 'A glamour drug that was once a celebrity and media choice has become cheaper and more accessible.' Mike Goodman, director of the UK drugs advice line Release agreed, pointing out that clubs where cocaine was popular also did a roaring trade in champagne: 'It's all linked to lifestyle,' he said. 'People have got more money, cocaine is cheaper. You can get it for £40 [$60] a gram, which people will club together and buy to share between them on a Saturday night.'

The UN's *Global Illicit Drug Trends* report for 2001 confirms a rising trend in western Europe, South and Central America, South Africa and Australia. What is termed 'occasional' cocaine use has stabilized in the USA (the world's largest market) at 1.7 per cent of the population aged 12 and over. This is a reduction of two-thirds on the 1985 level. Even so, when 'hardcore' (ie at least weekly) users are counted there are currently 6.6 million people, or 3 per cent of the entire US population, who take cocaine. Spin the numbers however you will, this is not a drug bound for oblivion.

CHARLIE: A POTTED BIOGRAPHY

So where and why do people take cocaine? How can cocaine culture be defined in the 21st century? To break down the big picture, it's worth separating South American chewers (coca leaf) from snorters (powder coke), smokers (crack cocaine or 'freebase'), mainliners (injected coke solution) and drinkers (usually coke dissolved in alcohol). For reasons that will become clearer in the crack section below, it's the chewers and snorters who mostly get along without setting up home in the gutter. Mainliners and drinkers are rarer breeds and are probably flirting with trouble. Regular crack smokers generally claim they're not addicted. Generally, they're lying.

CHEWERS AND SNORTERS

Coca leaf chewing has been going on for thousands of years in South America and only very rarely causes social or health problems. Powder coke has been around in the West for about 120 years and doesn't necessarily affect a user's health. That's not to say it is either safe or harmless. If you've got the money and the lifestyle that allow you to snort ten lines a day (a line is about one-twentieth of a gram or two-hundredths of an ounce) you're fast-tracking towards a serious habit. But a lot of users don't do cocaine this way. They'll take a line or two at a party or during a night out clubbing, and they won't touch it during the week. This is one reason why comparatively few coke and ecstasy users end up in hospital emergency departments.

SMOKERS

Freebase and crack cocaine are more recent derivatives of the drug and those that plan to fish in these waters need to be much more careful. When a drug is smoked, it reaches the brain in under four seconds. Recent research suggests that this speed of delivery greatly boosts cocaine's addictive qualities and leads to the 'bingeing' so common among crack and freebase addicts.

WHO IS THIS BOOK FOR?

This book is for users, their friends and parents, and anyone interested in a balanced perspective of cocaine in today's world. It looks at the drug's curious history, its links with music and showbusiness, fashion and pop culture. It explores the extraordinary underworld dealings of drug lords, traffickers and smugglers, and explains why crack has emerged as a key factor in street crime and gang warfare. It considers the power politics that drive world coca leaf production, and the terrible poverty that afflicts either end of the trade, from growers to consumers. Above all, it explains the science of cocaine addiction, the health implications and ways in which users can minimize risk.

If you're doing cocaine, or you know someone who is, then it's worth taking a look.

'Once I started, other people got to hear, and that type of thing, it escalates very quickly ... I was on the club scene every week, meeting different people, socializing. People come saying, "Can you get me some?" And as soon as it started – phew! – it got out of control, really.'

– Convicted 21-year-old woman recalling how she became
a clubland cocaine dealer, UK Home Office study, 2001

SOMETHING FOR THE WEEKEND?

For the best part of a century cocaine has been the music lover's drug of choice. The link dates back to the early American jazz and blues scene but it re-emerged strongly in popular culture with the *Easy Rider* generation of the late 1960s, the fast-living rockers of the 1970s and the new romantics of the 1980s. More recently, it has permeated clubland where, though ecstasy remains the market leader, a core of older clubbers see coke as more sophisticated and manageable.

With a rush lasting barely 40 minutes party lovers know they can pep themselves up on the dance floor and come down whenever they need to resume normal service. As one regular user of both drugs explained, 'With ecstasy you spend 15 hours grinning at everyone. With C [coke] you can buy a £20 [$30] half-gram special and just dip in and out of your emotions.'

Ed Jaram, editor of the British-based Internet club magazine *Spaced*, says that price is also a factor in the drug divide among the country's 1.5 million regular clubbers. 'There is some resistance to powder coke on the scene,' he says. 'First, it's more expensive and so tends to be used by an older, more affluent crowd. Second, clubbers want to know what they're buying. With pills you can see a stamp and you pretty much know what you've got. But with coke you could be buying speed or even talcum powder. You don't know until you try it.

Violence in the cocaine trade has seen a huge increase in the number of US Drug Enforcement Administration officers licensed to carry guns and make arrests. Between 1998 and 2000, the number rose by 26 per cent to 4,161. US Department of Justice, July 2001

'As a currency in clubs I don't think coke will ever overtake ecstasy, although a lot of people are starting to combine the two. For sure, everyone on the dance floor looks like they've been fuelled by the same ecstasy dealer but, chances are, there'll be quite a few older clubbers in there using coke or taking it cocktail style with Es.

'There's a good reason for this. If you want to stay up dancing all night you can take a load of pills but you'll get in a real mess. Older clubbers don't particularly enjoy swallowing six or seven pills and stumbling around mashed up and incoherent. That's more a teenage scene, which goes alongside binge drinking. Instead they take cocaine for kicks, or simply for energy. It's just a different approach.

'Cocaine is not perceived as a problem. Clubbers live for weekend culture and because of this they don't associate it with day-to-day life. The association is going out and having one night of being completely trashed. Then it's back to the work-a-day week. Given that pattern of use, cocaine can be managed. Crack is very different but then crack hardly features at all in clubland.'

CLUBBERS' DELIGHT

London is the unchallenged club capital of Britain on the basis that there are so damn many of them. They do different styles on different days, which means you can groove away to the easy listening of Karen Carpenter and Englebert Humperdinck and return the following night to a thrashing techno mêlée of leather and fetishwear. Then there's all the stops in between – jungle, hip-hop, rap, contemporary soul, R&B, salsa, Latin, nosebleed, trance, hardcore techno and house. Oh, and Eurohouse. And handbag house. Need I go on?

Club nights are essentially multimedia fashion statements. The demonic lighting effects with their white flashes and eerie green glows, the dancers silhouetted against the strobes, the huge, full-on drum beats, the outrageous DJs playing tracks simultaneously, the muscle-bound bodies, the day-glo green T-shirts, the white leather underwear — if it's remotely cool, it's on show. And, of course, drugs are part of this show, despite the body searches on the door and the official warning words from police and proprietors.

'Cocaine and ecstasy use is now so widespread, and so accepted by promoters and the police, that the legal position isn't much of a talking point,' says Jaram. Everyone has their own view but it is taken for granted in Britain that you can go to a club and do drugs and nobody is going to mind.

'Promoters and owners are very, very tolerant towards this lifestyle. You can buy your stuff, take it in and do it, and you know you're not going to get thrown out. The question of legalization doesn't arise because you're using drugs anyway without hassle.

'As a general rule clubbers are aware of the dangers they face. This is much more important to them than whether some politician somewhere says a drug is legal or not. There certainly isn't the kind of repression found in, say, New York where clubs are influenced by a zero tolerance attitude to anything perceived as crime.'

REDUCING THE RISKS?

This may be true, although the British government is beaming out some confused signals. In March 2002 the Home Office launched a booklet entitled *Safer Clubbing*. This called for more effort to stop weapons being smuggled past doormen (see the later section on cocaine and street crime) but also acknowledged that coke and ecstasy were part of the club scene. The booklet urged proprietors to provide more drinking water, cut out overcrowding and overheating, improve ventilation, train staff to spot the effects of intoxication and offer a 'calm environment' where users can chill out or get treatment.

'If we cannot stop them from taking drugs then we must be prepared to take steps to reduce the harm that they may cause themselves,' said Bob Ainsworth, Home Office minister. 'Unfortunately, for many young club-goers, illegal drug use has become an integral part of their night out. Club owners and dance promoters have a duty to make sure that they have done everything possible to reduce the risks faced by the young people who are their paying customers. We have to recognize that some clubbers will continue to ignore the risks and carry on taking dangerous drugs.'

This is fine and dandy, except the Home Office also announced proposals for tough new laws aimed at jailing proprietors and nightclub managers who knowingly allow 'dance scene' drugs like cocaine to be consumed on their premises. At the very least, this is a contradiction in policy. The message to clubs is: 'Keep drug users safe when they're on your premises. And by the way, don't let them in at all.'

A REAL GROWTH INDUSTRY

According to a Home Office study published in 2001 – *Middle Market Drug Distribution*, by Geoffrey Pearson (Goldsmiths College) and Dick Hobbs (University of London) – the clubbing scene is 'a modern system of fraternity that can facilitate drug networks and highly accelerated drug dealing careers'. Pearson and Hobbs interviewed prisoners who started by selling a few tablets around the dance scene and progressed within months to become 'serious middle market drugs brokers'.

One 21-year-old woman told them: 'Once I started, other people got to hear, and that type of thing, it escalates very quickly ... I was on the club scene every week, meeting different people, socializing. People come saying, "Can you get me some?" And as soon as it started – phew! – it got out of control, really.'

A 30-year-old man explained how in a typical weekend he would shift 2,500 ecstasy pills, 4kg (9lb) of marijuana, 110g (4oz) of cocaine and various quantities of speed and LSD. He started selling to friends, then friends of friends and a network quickly built up. 'Eventually you've got other people who want to start dealing and then dealers buy from you and it's a sky rocket before you even know it. I don't agree with selling in clubs, it's more like pushing drugs ... I didn't push drugs at all. I did a social thing for friends and then it just got bigger.' Networking is the lifeblood of the cocaine dealer. The sharper ones will sell you a few lines and then invite you to a party to share them. If you run out – no problem: there's plenty more for sale.

MADDY'S STORY

Maddy* discovered this when she began exploring London's gay scene early in 2001. Then a 22-year-old student of English and Drama, she started work in a lesbian bar in central London, trying an occasional line out of interest. Until then she'd avoided drugs completely.

'I had very conservative views of drugs,' she told me. 'I barely drank alcohol until after I was 18 and even when I went to uni I was a total lightweight. I softened up when I took speed to help me work all night on essays. Then I had a couple of lines at a New Year's Eve 2001 party, decided I liked it and found it easy to buy. My habit progressed very quickly from there. I thought, "Wow I really fit in." I'm gay and I grew up in a small town that was homophobic and racist, and I used to go to a gay pub from the age of 16, just to escape.

'If you drink on the gay scene in London [cocaine use] is absolutely rife, it really is. If you go into any toilet cubicle and wipe your hand along the back of the cistern I will guarantee you'll get some powder coke off it. When everybody around you is doing it you think, "Hey, this stuff can't be

> An ongoing study of UK student drug use by Professor Howard Parker of Manchester University found a 400 per cent increase in the number who had tried cocaine. He discovered a 'normalization' of cocaine use and told the *Observer* newspaper, 'I have no doubt that cocaine is becoming the drug of choice, after cannabis.' *Observer*, 22 April 2001

so bad." We'd all go out clubbing and I'd do about nine lines a night and stay up till 5 or 6am.

'After a while, though, people work out what you're about and you become a magnet to dealers. All the gay guys in the pub – people I'd just been good mates with – they began inviting me back to parties. These were the same guys who supplied me. Some really took the piss. They'd

* Some details have been changed to protect Maddy's anonymity

sell to me then invite me somewhere because they knew I'd got coke on me. It's a great way for dealers to get free lines for the night!

'Cocaine was fun for about four months but then I'd come home from parties and find I'd still got some left. I wouldn't be able to leave it alone. I'd sit and do it on my own and play on the PlayStation, like out of my face. That's when you start thinking, "Is this really such a sociable drug?"

'Things came to a head when I started using a new dealer. The stuff he gave me was much purer than anything I'd had before and it was too much for me. It would upset my stomach, I got really paranoid; buzzing so much I didn't know what to do with myself. It wasn't nice but it was addictive. I started buying more and more. I went from buying one gram at a time to three grams. That would be for a big binge over 24 hours. I would seek out others who were into it so that I had an excuse.'

Maddy is clean of coke now. She's moved to a provincial English city, keeps in touch with the local drugs project and has a steady job. The thought of cocaine fills her with neither temptation nor bitterness. 'Looking back, despite all the problems I've had with cocaine, I still think that in the right circumstances it's a fun drug. It's certainly a lot safer than some other substances on the street. I've had some really wild nights with it, no question.'

AMERICA ON LINE

London's bar and club cocaine culture is rarely troubled by the law. Police busts aimed at users (as opposed to dealers) are rare. However, across the pond in New York there is a much more repressive attitude towards recreational drugs, so far with little deterrent effect. One correspondent working in the Big Apple for a British national newspaper during the 1990s described cocaine as 'the ultimate night-out accessory'. He was not a user but came to regard it as no different to alcohol and tobacco. 'In some ways it's more socially acceptable than both,' he says. 'You get it in little white home-made envelopes, which somehow seems a nice personal touch.

'It can be a pretty undignified method of consumption – bending over a bog seat and sniffing – but once that's out of the way then the result is attractive. Cocaine doesn't poison other people, like tobacco smoke, and it doesn't make your drinking companion vomit 12 lagers over you. If you're a club regular, or a stock trader, or in the media then coke comes with the territory. The police keep publicizing these big drugs clampdowns but most New Yorkers on the scene don't even notice. If anything, cocaine is getting easier to buy.'

The correspondent recalled how UK journalists based in New York during the 1970s – 'they could all have drunk for Britain' – used to be given a line or two to sober them up. The Brit hack pack would frequent a writers' and musicians' bar in Greenwich Village called the Bells of Hell. Whenever the atmosphere got too tasty a member of the bar staff would call offenders into the kitchen, cut some lines with a credit card and offer the alternatives of snorting it or leaving the premises. Invariably they took a snort.

Today, corporate America remains awash with the drug. There's a dealers' paradise on South Beach, Miami, Florida, every March when thousands of house, techno and electronic music fans descend for the annual Winter Music Conference. This is supposed to unearth strange new beats and cutting-edge artists, but more recently it has become an exercise in branding, marketing and corporate focus groups. Where full-on music company executives meet the house crowd you can bet your deck blender that cocaine supplies will be somewhere nearby. Usually in a large truck.

In its report of the 2002 South Beach shindig, the Internet mag *wired.com* quoted a travel executive reminiscing about a party the previous year, held on a music multinational's rooftop reception area. 'If it hadn't been so windy,' he recalls wistfully, 'people would have been doing lines off each others' shoulders.'

This is only just an exaggeration. Cocaine powers the music business – not just the dance scene – and has done for much of the 20th century. When in 2001 the British rock music TV channel VH1 ran a poster advertising campaign, it used a photo of three children's drinking straws alongside a rolled-up banknote apparently tipped with white powder. The copy read: 'VH1. Music TV that's not for kids.'

When the channel was hauled before the Advertising Standards Authority (ASA) it accepted that the ad was a bit risqué while insisting that the strange white powder was in fact a printing error. This ranks among the truly great caught-in-possession excuses: 'What you're looking at there officer, that's a printing error.' VH1's stronger argument – namely that you can't ignore the sex, drugs and rock'n'roll heritage of popular music – failed to persuade the watchdog. The ASA banned the poster on the grounds that it implied drug taking was acceptable. Strange when you think that for at least three decades the songwriters who drive youth culture have been telling the world that drugs are cool.

MUSIC, FASHION, WORK … AND A LINE FOR CELEBRITIES

In 1975, the American rock legend JJ Cale wrote the song 'Cocaine'. It's inconceivable that you don't know the lyrics but here's a brief reminder anyway:

> 'If you wanna hang out you've got to take her out – cocaine
> If you wanna get down, down on the ground – cocaine
> She don't lie, she don't lie, she don't lie – cocaine'

Now, in some respects ol' JJ has got a lot to answer for. If it hadn't been for him then Eric Clapton would never have done a cover version. And if Clapton hadn't pumped up the volume we'd all have been spared years of listening to late-night disco and wedding party revellers singing along loudly, drunkenly and hopelessly out of tune. If you're looking for a real cocaine scandal this is it. But, let's face it, no government is ever going to ban Clapton. It's only a question of time before he gets a knighthood.

According to a survey by the Partnership for a Drug Free America (27 November 2000), 2.4 million American teenagers have tried cocaine or crack. This is 10 per cent of the teen population, up by 1 per cent on the previous year and up significantly on 1993.

The song became an anthem for the cocaine boom of the 1970s and reinforced the tabloid press view that all filthy-rotten-rich rock stars were on the stuff. As generalizations go, this one was on the button. It didn't apply so much to the punk movement mind, because punks saw cocaine as a bourgeois affectation, completely unnecessary when you could pop speed and ecstasy.

Still, over the last three decades, your typical pop star seems to have been at least an occasional coke-head. Songs like Black Sabbath's 'Snowblind' or Suede's 'We Are The Pigs', written after an experience of coke-induced paranoia according to the band's Brett Anderson, kept cocaine up there as a fashion drug. There were some truly great lines – no, let's call them lyrics – from the 1990s. In the Oasis track 'What's The Story ...', Noel Gallagher wrote: 'All your dreams are made when you're chained to a mirror and a razor blade.'

CHARLIE'S WITH THE BAND...

Here, courtesy of the British website studentUK.com, are a few more reflections from the stars and industry execs who were sniffing around at the time. For the benefit of the uninitiated, razors or credit cards are commonly used to chop cocaine into a fine powder and arrange it into lines. Mirrors are used as a chopping surface because they ensure very little waste.

'You get up in the morning, surrounded by empty bottles, and the mirror's covered in smears of cocaine and the first thing you do is lick the mirror' – Elton John recalling the drug days of his early career in the 1970s (according to John's biographer Philip Norman the singer got such a megalomanic buzz from the drug that he once asked aides to 'turn down the wind' because the sound of swaying trees was bothering him)

'Cocaine is a very spiteful bedfellow. If you want to lose all the friends and relationships you ever held dear, that's the drug to do it with' – David Bowie, in his 'Thin White Duke' phase

'I take cocaine. Big fucking deal' – Noel Gallagher, Oasis

'There's a fucking blizzard of cocaine in London at the moment and I hate it. It's stupid. Everyone's become so blasé, thinking they're so ironic and witty and wandering around with that stupid fucking cokey confidence. Wankers. I did it, but I can't say I was a cocaine addict' – Damon Albarn, Blur, speaking in 1996

> *'By the time I was 23 I was addicted but it didn't seem to matter in*
> *our business. No one thought it was unusual to be up all night doing*
> *lines of coke'* – Alan McGee, head of Creation Records

As you can see, cocaine was – and still is – ingrained in music culture. Sir Paul McCartney tried it when he was writing The Beatles *Sgt. Pepper's Lonely Hearts Club Band* album in 1966. He got the drug from art gallery dealer Robert Fraser (one of the bastions of trendy London in the 1960s) who was in turn supplied by an American designer. In a biography entitled *Groovy Bob*, Harriet Vyner tells how Fraser also introduced The Rolling Stones to coke, along with a beautiful young member of their circle called Marianne Faithfull.

Apparently when Marianne was offered her first line she didn't know the etiquette and snorted in one go everything that Fraser had laid out. At least she didn't go the way of lead guitarist Ronnie Wood, widely reported to have destroyed part of his nose through overuse of the drug (see Danniella Westbrook, p25). It was said that Wood woke up one morning to discover that he could see the bathroom sink through the the top of his hooter.

During the 1970s, when rock'n'roll excesses were attaining new heights, rumours circulated about a new method of taking cocaine that wouldn't give you a rotten proboscis. The drug can be absorbed into the blood through any membrane (this is why it's sometimes rubbed on gums) and, inevitably, imaginative types explored a variety of techniques. Apparently the rock stars' 'special' involved anal administration, colloquially known as gak blowing, and gossip abounded about bands with a resident gak blower on their tour bus. It's unclear whether knee-pads were provided. If you want to know exactly how gak blowing is done then ask someone else; the research budget on this book is way too low.

Doing cocaine is now practically expected in the music business. We're not quite at the point where record company executives give superstars a roasting on the grounds that they should snort – or perhaps gak – more lines, but it can't be far off. Just look at Robbie Williams, for whom coke has arguably been career enhancing.

During his years with Take That, Williams signed up to the scrupulously controlled sparkly clean image demanded by record label bosses. Then in June 1995 he threw his toys out of his cot and headed for the Glastonbury rock festival with Oasis. As he later told music magazine *Select*, he tried 'every drug except heroin'. Since then, Williams has deservedly achieved superstar status – both for his songwriting and singing. As quickly as he took up his bad boy image he dumped it, attending a rehab centre, slimming down and staying clean of drugs.

Some musical movements became synonymous with cocaine. In the early 1980s the new romantics dominated British pop, with synthetically produced bands spawning outrageous fashion chic. The founder of this movement was Steve Strange, owner of the Covent Garden nightclub Blitz, who would stand at the door in leather jodhpurs and German SS-style overcoat deciding who was original and stylish enough to be let in. He once famously turned away Jagger, allegedly holding a mirror up to the wrinkly star's face and asking, 'Would you let yourself in?' Strange denies this, insisting the place was simply full. But it made a cracking piece for the tabloids.

Strange founded one of the first new romantic bands, Visage, co-writing the mega-hit 'Fade To Grey' in 1980 with Midge Ure. Writing in the *Mail On Sunday* in March 2002 he recalls how until this point his only vice had been drink, which he used to overcome his natural shyness at being Blitz's centre of attention. After Visage, everything changed.

'The pop business was different,' he wrote. 'Wherever I went, cocaine was on offer. There was always an accommodating dealer on hand cutting up lines of white powder. Soon I was using so much cocaine, and sharing so much, that I had a courier permanently on stand-by to collect fresh supplies. It was as much a part of the music industry as guitars and drums.'

COKE ON THE CATWALK

Cocaine was, at the same time, becoming the unspoken accessory of fashion modelling. There are obvious reasons for this. Like pop stars, models need to keep a good handle on their image. You can't shimmy down a catwalk with puncture marks in your arms or a big gurney grin shaped by too much ecstasy the night before. You can't be drunk because it's not conducive to moving in straight lines. Amphetamines are out because, hell, you'd do the

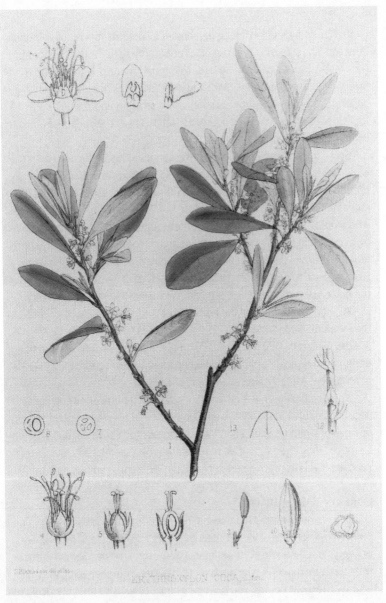

Illustration of the coca plant (*Erythroxylon coca*), the source of cocaine, after an engraving by Blair in *Medicinal Plants* (London, 1880).

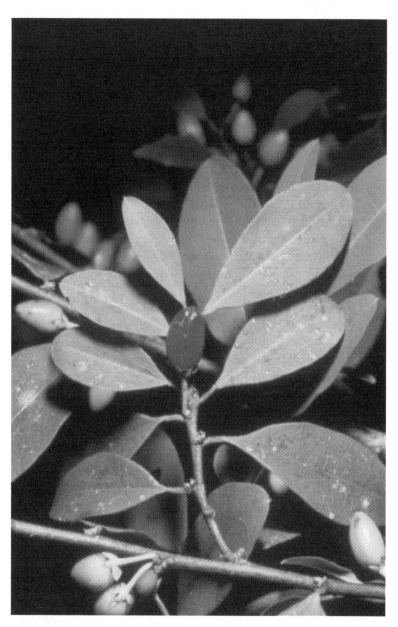

The fruit and leaves of *Erythroxylon coca*.

catwalk in a personal best of 7.2 seconds. What you need is a drug that gets your eyes sparkling (by restricting the blood supply to them) and your confidence zooming. Just a little make-up for the mind.

Strange's *Mail On Sunday* article coincided with a frenzy of media interest in cocaine in general and the fashion business in particular. The catalyst for this was a decision by 'supermodel' Naomi Campbell to sue the London-based *Mirror* newspaper for compensation after it revealed that she was receiving therapy for drug abuse and had attended Narcotics Anonymous meetings. Campbell won rather a pyrrhic victory, receiving only £3,500 ($5,070) on a somewhat technical legal argument. She was also accused by the High Court judge of lying under oath.

The evidence was, as always in these cases, much more interesting than the outcome. In a written statement, *Mirror* editor Piers Morgan argued that publication was justified because Campbell had publicly denied her addiction to drugs while committing a serious offence 'by possessing and using a Class A drug – cocaine – over a period of years'.

The *Mirror*'s barrister, Desmond Browne, QC, asked her: 'If you make a bargain with fame to achieve success you have to live with the consequences and not whine about it.'

Campbell replied: 'I am a drug addict. I will always be an addict. Once an addict always an addict. I am not ashamed of it because I am in recovery.' Of the *Mirror* she said: 'They knew nothing about recovery or treatment. They knew nothing about the harm they could have done me.' Then, looking directly at Browne she added, 'And neither do you understand recovery, by the way, as it isn't as simple as you think it is. It's a lifelong process.'

Morgan, for his part, rejected any suggestion that he had run the story recklessly. 'We could have done a come-on, asking people who had snorted coke with her to come forward, but we didn't,' he insisted. 'It was a very sympathetic article and I am amazed she took such exception.'

Other models have spoken less reluctantly about the effect of cocaine on their lives. The Californian-born icon Carre Otis, who in the 1990s became the face of Calvin Klein, admitted in a 2002 interview with the London *Sunday Times* that she used the drug to help maintain her skeletal figure. She is now clean and an attractively healthy 'plus-size' (as they euphemistically term it in the clothes-horse business).

'The only way that I have ever been a size 10 was when I starved myself,' she said. 'Or I was doing huge amounts of cocaine or just drinking and not eating. That's the only time I have ever been really skinny.' For Otis, use of the drug carried a terrible history. Aged just 15 she had been dating the son of a Californian politician when the boy lost a soccer match, got himself high on cocaine and blew his brains out. The suicide note was addressed to her.

When Otis later realised her potential as a model she felt a confusing sensation of power combined with self-loathing. 'I was fasting, taking diet pills, laxatives, Dexedrine and all sorts of other drugs including cocaine and alcohol. I was also cutting myself. It was really an attempt to have some control over a life that was out of control. The only thing I could control [was] what I did with my body, what went in my mouth. I was the controller of the pain.'

THE SOCIALITE'S CHUM

In fact, as she later realised, cocaine was the controller of the pain. This was also the experience of queen of the 'It' Girls, Tara Palmer-Tomkinson, who in 1990s Britain became the darling of the popular press – proper posh totty according to the red-top papers. Palmer-Tomkinson's forte was partying and being outrageous – that and the fact that her family knew Prince Charles very well.

From the moment she was photographed giving HRH a quick kiss in the Swiss ski resort of Klosters, Tara was on the A-list for every celebrity bash, PR launch and fashion show in town. Partying was her chosen career and, as she put it, 'Daddy had always told me to do my best in whatever I chose to do and I didn't want to disappoint.'

In an article for the *Daily Mail*'s *Weekend* magazine (16 March 2002) she writes: 'As an It Girl it was simply my job to amuse. I took the role very seriously. I always tried to entertain – to sing for my supper. And sadly, this is how I started to rely on cocaine.

'...It seemed to give me the energy and the confidence I needed to discourse brilliantly with people from all walks of life. To begin with, I took it before an evening out but the habit escalated and soon I couldn't face the world without it. At the same time I realised that the confidence it gave me was illusory. Cocaine began to eat away at my self-esteem. It took away my natural vivacity and made me restless and paranoid. I was still going to three parties a night and I could never sit still.'

She goes on to describe the cringe-makingly embarrassing episode of her 27th birthday party. There was a James Bond theme and a suitably coked-up Tara was photographed at the door dressed in bikini, stiletto boots and a snorkel. She was supposed to be Ursula Andress except that, in that get-up, she could have frightened Dr No to death without troubling 007.

'The posse of hangers-on that was my drug-taking coterie encouraged this wild behaviour,' she wrote. 'Meanwhile, my true friends and family were desperately worried. As my cocaine habit grew, my drinking increased. I became deceitful and self-obsessed. Life stopped being frivolous and fun.' She tried to fight this by returning regularly to the family home in Hampshire for drug-free recuperation. But when she got back to London she got back to cocaine.

ACTING UP

It was the kind of self-deception nightmare succinctly summed up by American actor/director and one-time three-grams-a-day coke user Dennis Hopper. Even when he stopped drinking in 1983 and began attending Alcoholics Anonymous it took him another year to finally kiss goodbye to cocaine.

'I would turn up at meetings, saying "I'm an alcoholic" with half an ounce of cocaine in my pocket,' he told the London *Daily Telegraph* (29 January 2001). 'And I wouldn't smoke grass, or use any downers or anything because that was going to take me over the edge. I mean, how crazy am I? So, finally, I just burned out again, and the radio was talking to me and the electric wires – boy, I was out of it. So if anybody has any doubts about cocaine – cocaine is just as bad on its own without any help from anything else.'

To Palmer-Tomkinson's credit she has also fought her way clean via a spell at a rehab clinic – Meadows, near Wickenburg, Arizona – and dumped the dealers and users who circled her every move. She has since re-launched her journalistic career and does charity work for organizations such as Chemical Dependency. Self-evidently, cocaine never took away her looks.

SNOW ON THE SMALL SCREEN

The *EastEnders* soap actress Danniella Westbrook was less fortunate. Little known outside the UK, her cocaine habit produced a powerful reminder of how heavy use of the drug can break down human tissue. Photographs of her taken during 2000 showed how her septum (the part of her nose between the nostrils) had vanished, her single nasal orifice a cruel parody of the star's former beauty. This is a condition that can be rectified by plastic surgery, but it shattered her career – at least temporarily.

Westbrook's rumoured £300-a-day ($435) habit revealed an astonishing level of addiction for a woman still in her mid-twenties and is untypical of most users. As the journalist and author Julie Burchill put it later: 'I just don't know how she did it. Between 1986 and 1996 I must have put enough toot up my admittedly sizeable snout to stun the entire Colombian armed forces and still it sits there, Romanesque and proud, all too bloody solid actually.'

Other British celebrities have lived to regret cocaine's allure for different reasons. John Alford, a star of the hit TV fire service drama *London's Burning*, was jailed for nine months and lost his £120,000-a-year ($175,000) role after he was caught selling the drug to an undercover reporter. It took four years for him to claw his way back into a minor TV role. But the biggest scandal to hit British television came in March 2001 when Stuart Lubbock, a party guest at the Essex home of TV presenter and comedian Michael Barrymore, was found dead in the star's swimming pool.

In a TV interview with the journalist Martin Bashir, Barrymore denied allegations that he had given cocaine to his guests and said he had merely smoked cannabis on the night, but he also admitted: 'Any time I wasn't working I would immediately start drinking and taking pills just to get me away. I took drugs as well. I smoked pot, [took] cocaine, Es, speed, anything.' After a year-long investigation, Essex police announced that no further action would be taken. Barrymore escaped with an arrest and caution for possession of cannabis and allowing his home to be used for smoking the drug.

AMERICAN HIGH
America, though, remains the spiritual home of the cocaine scandal. Perhaps the best known involved the comedian Richard Pryor, who on 9 June 1980 had just finished a freebase smoking binge (still a strange concept to most Americans) when he decided to round things off by drinking the high-percentage-proof rum swilling around his waterpipe. After five days non-stop freebasing Pryor was pretty much shot to shreds and he spilled the rum down his highly flammable nylon shirt. Then he decided to light a cigarette, ignited the fumes as well and effectively blew himself up. He needed months of burns treatment but was still able to joke to an audience how he 'did the 100-yard dash in 4.3'.

Pryor was lucky. Not so fellow comedian John Belushi. He was lured by the intrinsically dangerous 'speedball' cocktail of heroin and cocaine, an upper-downer combination that has fascinated habitual drug users for much of the 20th century. The two drugs combine extremely well in terms of their buzz, although the physical effect has been likened to driving at maximum revs with the brakes screaming. For Belushi, loved by millions as the anarchic star of the cult movie *The Blues Brothers*, it was one ride too many. He died in March 1982 of a speedball overdose.

FRIEND OF THE FAMOUS
Truth is, the link between cocaine and celebrities has become so well established over the last two decades that its use is now an open secret. When the British comedienne Caroline Aherne – aka Mrs Merton – compered the 1997 Brit Awards her coke quip got the biggest laugh of the night: 'Does anyone know where Charlie is?' she pleaded with the audience. 'Everyone backstage has been asking for him.'

Aherne's gag was aimed not only at the household names in front of camera. Use of cocaine has become a social ritual cherished by the media executives who create those same stars. It's now so commonplace that discretion is almost a dirty word in some quarters of TV land.

THE PROFESSIONAL TOUCH

During the research for this book I spoke to a handful of professional people who I knew to be occasional users. One MP's aide assured me that 'California cornflakes' were certainly consumed around the House of Commons – and not only at breakfast time. But he didn't want to talk about it, even off the record. 'People might try to work out who I am,' he said. 'In politics, if you're caught dabbling in drugs it's still a career death sentence.'

It was the same story with a barrister, who saw coke as an essential 'heart-starter' for his openings in tricky cases, a mid-level banker, who revealed it was *de rigueur* in City toilets following heavy boozing sessions, a female PR executive who does cocaine with her pals over lunch at a West Kensington, London, restaurant, and a doctor who regards it as 'bloody essential' towards the

In 1999 an analysis of American males arrested by the Drug Enforcement Administration in 34 US cities revealed an average of 32.4 per cent testing positive for cocaine. This was only marginally lower than marijuana (39.9 per cent) and more than four times the number taking opiates such as heroin (7.4 per cent) and methamphetamine (7.3 per cent).

end of 48-hour shifts. All these people said they took powder cocaine either on their own or among small, select groups of friends or colleagues. While they didn't see coke use as remotely troubling, they were concerned about the risk of personal exposure.

Fair enough. At least my BBC contact didn't let me down. When I told her of my difficulties in getting interviews – even unattributable ones – she laughed out loud. 'I suppose the Beeb could have a witch-hunt,' she said. 'But I doubt they'd even care. If they really cared they'd have sacked a whole swathe of middle and senior management years ago. I cannot stress enough to you that snorting a line of coke is considered totally unremarkable behaviour at the BBC.'

The woman, a young and highly regarded programme maker, is not a cocaine user herself and admits that she was incredibly naïve when in 1992 she was offered a line by an award-winning executive in his office. 'I hadn't a clue what he was talking about,' she said. 'Then he just laid this stuff out on his desk, pulled a short drinking straw out of a drawer and sniffed it up.

'I was very new at the time and a bit shocked that he would do this in front of a junior colleague he'd hardly met. I thought that perhaps he was trying to impress me. Over the years I've come to realise that he wasn't. For him it was like lighting a cigarette or pouring a cup of coffee. It was an act not even considered worthy of comment.

'Cocaine use is considered absolutely fine at TV launch parties or media receptions where everyone knows everyone, and everyone knows that everyone else is doing it. There really is no discretion. But there is a recognition that where outsiders are mixing with you, you should be a bit more careful.

'The problem occurs when people get horrendously drunk, lose that sense of caution and feel the need for a line. I remember being taken to a major awards ceremony at some warehouse place in north London. There was senior management around because various programmes had done well. Everybody was in the mood to celebrate and it was snowing cocaine in the toilets.

'By the end of the evening people weren't even bothering to go to the loo. Most of the non-media types had pulled out and cocaine was being laid out on the tables and shared among everyone who wanted it. There was a general feeling afterwards that things had gone a bit too far. The trouble is, that when cocaine is as familiar as the office furniture nobody ever says "C'mon guys, be careful." It just doesn't occur to them.

I will say that my only experience with cocaine involved having sex with a colleague who'd taken it. It was absolutely wonderful because I've never known a man who could manage sex three times without a break.'

Toby Young, one of the few national newspaper journalists willing to talk openly about his coke use, tells how he once appeared on a BBC current affairs programme to discuss Home Office statistics about cocaine-related deaths. Just before going on he mentioned conspiratorially to the producer how he'd bought along his forensic testing kit. Would she mind if he gave the studio lavatories a quick once over? The producer giggled nervously. 'Only joking,' said Young.

In an article for the *Observer* (18 November 2001), Young also criticized the directors of the Groucho Club, London's foremost media den, for kicking him out. His crime was to write about providing cocaine for two of the trendiest names in British art – Damien Hirst and Keith Allen – during a photo shoot at the Groucho. Neither man has ever tried to hide his appreciation of illegal drugs and Hirst has spoken openly about his own cocaine use in a compilation of interviews entitled *On The Way To Work*.

'I didn't think the Groucho would mind if I wrote about this,' recalls Young. 'After all, it's hardly a state secret that people occasionally take cocaine in the club. On the contrary, if Osama bin Laden sent a suspicious-looking envelope full of white powder to 45 Dean Street, it would be up someone's nose in 30 seconds.' Touché. Lest the Groucho feels unfairly singled out over this episode, let's not forget that some of the best establishments in the capital experience a regular sprinkling of joy powder. A forensic survey commissioned by the *London Evening Standard* found traces at the Savoy Hotel, the Ritz and even the Royal Opera House. So, that's how they hit the high notes.

There are some great urban myths about cocaine and the chattering classes. Actually, they probably aren't myths. On Wall Street, Gordon Gecko types still carry around solid gold and silver razor blades to cut lines. The exclusive jeweller Tiffany is said to have withdrawn sales of silver cocktail straws because they are a fashion icon for coke-heads. Certain west London eateries are rumoured to provide horizontal mirrors in private rooms. Now, apart from checking out your double chin, what possible practical use might these have?

Then there are the glass-fronted pictures in hotel suites, which bear a white smear. This is supposedly the tell-tale mark of the cocaine user who has removed the picture, laid it flat, cut and snorted his coke and wiped a finger over the precious white remnants of powder to rub into his gums. Cocaine culture is so ritualistic at times.

However at that bastion of middle-class ritual – the private London dinner party – it is apparently consumed with no more ceremony than a glass of port or after-dinner mint. Some hostesses are said to arrange it as a kind of hors-d'œuvre on silver platters or china plates. Or it can be found on the mantelpiece, a simple accessory to social intercourse; to be taken, or not, without comment. This may all be anecdotal stuff but, among the UK's professional classes, the notion that cocaine is as accessible as chocolate lollies in the Willie Wonka factory is hard to dispute.

As Ed Jaram at *Spaced* says, 'Coke has become part of the metropolitan bar culture. [It] is really taking off, particularly in boom areas like Shoreditch [north London]. There are a lot of professional people in their twenties and thirties hanging out in these places at lunchtime and after work. They've got disposable income and easy access to suppliers. For them cocaine is an obvious drug of choice because they can use it without affecting their work.'

It seems to affect the crime rate though.

STREET CRIME

Cocaine and crime are soulmates. Especially in western cities. Nowhere is this more true than London, which in 2001 saw an explosion in inter-gang violence and street crime apparently caused by crack addicts desperate for some rocks. The major crack suppliers in Britain are Jamaican or of Jamaican origin – often described as 'Yardie' gangs. They have Caribbean associates who arrange imports from Colombia while they act as wholesalers in overall control of UK and some European distribution. They are part of a worldwide trafficking operation (of which more later). They may also organize street dealing and sales to approved dealers.

According to the head of Scotland Yard's Flying Squad, Commander Alan Brown, Yardie-style gangsters are now the most violent and difficult criminals faced by British police. On 16 January 2002 he released figures showing 21 drug-related murders and 67 attempted murders in London the previous year. All but two of the capital's 32 boroughs (districts) had reported drug-linked crime and all but ten had seen shootings. In the previous fortnight police had logged the first two murders of the new year and a further 25 shootings. All of this was 'black-on-black' crime.

The figures for gun crime across England and Wales rose by 9 per cent in 2001 to 4,019 incidents. It's hard to know how much of this was linked to cocaine in particular and drugs in general, but police believe that a significant proportion is down to Yardie in-fighting and feuding. It is all uncannily similar to the extreme violence on the streets of Miami and New York in the 1980s when America woke up to its own crack epidemic (see Chapter 3).

One of the best-placed observers of that phenomenon was a doctor living and working in the Haight-Ashbury district of San Francisco. Dr David Smith had been to medical school there and studied for his graduate degree in pharmacology. He became interested in recreational drugs and specifically the way they were affecting young Americans eager to experiment. In June 1967 he set up the Haight-Ashbury Free Clinic (HAFC), providing free healthcare for drug patients. Today HAFC has 22 sites in the Bay Area and deals with 50,000 client visits a year. As past president of the American Society of Addiction Medicine, Smith knows his stuff. He remembers clearly the complacency he encountered in Britain when he tried to warn of a European coke'n'crime boom.

'I gave a lecture in London in the 1980s,' he said. 'One of the UK's leading experts on cocaine – I can't remember who now – was saying: "Look, we have no cocaine problem in England and we never will because our security at ports is so tight." I argued that if you have market demand, law enforcement alone will not stop it. To believe otherwise was really very naïve.

'What we'd been hearing from the Drug Enforcement Administration in the US was that the American crack cocaine market was becoming saturated. It was basically a loose cannon because the drug was so toxic – users either died or went crazy or got into downers like heroin or alcohol. This is why the Colombian cartels began marketing cocaine in southern Europe – particularly Spain – and Jamaica, and exchanging it for heroin.

'That drove the cocaine epidemic in Europe. I'm not into the "I told you so" philosophy but this is exactly as we predicted twenty years ago. We learnt by looking at broad cycles and understanding cocaine culture.

'At present around 80 per cent of people in the American criminal justice system have substance abuse problems. Only 5 per cent get treatment. If you're black and from a lower socio-economic class you have a ten times higher probability of becoming a felon than if you're white and middle class. If you're black you go to prison. If you're white you get treatment.

'Crack cocaine moving into the black culture is a major factor in this paradigm. At Haight-Ashbury we did a random medication study on amphetamine and crack cocaine. In the amphetamine study every one of the recruited patients turned out to be white. In the cocaine study every one was black.

'In San Francisco, methamphetamine is a big gay drug. But in many areas of America it is identified as a rural, white supremacist kind of drug whereas crack cocaine is seen as an urban, black drug – both of these have a high association with violence. Both act in a pharmacologically similar fashion in the brain, although methamphetamine is longer lasting. But the social and cultural aspect is very, very different. There seems to be a bigger rise in drug abuse, particularly speed labs, in rural America than in urban America. It is a very interesting phenomenon.

> **Almost one-third of Americans aged 12 or over believe that cocaine and crack is fairly or very easy to obtain. This figure showed a slight decline to around 30 per cent of the population in 2000.**
> Drug Enforcement Administration, Collective Statistics

'Crack cocaine has become an inner city, black, urban drug and methamphetamine has become a rural, white drug even though both have a high association with violence, even though both have a similar toxicity relative to heart attacks and strokes, and even though both are similar in terms of psychiatric toxicity.'

PSYCHIATRIC TOXICITY?

While London's crack cocaine gangs are not necessarily drug users themselves they certainly seem to be mad about guns. At Scotland Yard, Alan Brown heads the Operation Trident task force, which targets the big players. He has cited specific instances of how easily shootings are provoked in disputes about drugs, territory or 'respect'. Examples include:

- a sarcastic remark made by one black gangster about another's hairstyle
- a man treading on a gang leader's foot by mistake in a nightclub
- a nightclub bouncer refusing entry to a gang enforcer; the man returned with a gun and sprayed bullets at a queue waiting to enter the club; eight people were injured

■ a row between a party-goer and a DJ in which the DJ was shot dead; the bullet passed through a wall, killing a second man.

'There are clearly organizations in both Jamaica and [the UK] that have almost a business relationship for supply and retail,' said Brown. 'The drug and gun culture is producing an incredibly narcissistic generation of young criminals. Their reaction to any act of what they see as disrespect is extreme violence.'

Less than a month after Brown's media briefing in January 2002 there was one of the most overt assassination attempts yet in London's cocaine wars. In the early hours of 8 February, a Ford Mondeo was 'ambushed' by a silver Audi on the busy Wandsworth gyratory system. Someone in the Audi opened up with an Uzi machine pistol, also known as the 'spray and pray' because of its ability to deliver 600 rounds a minute. This is the Yardie enforcer's favourite weapon, lethal but notoriously hard to control.

On this occasion it punched ten bullet holes in the Mondeo, killing a male passenger. Desperate to escape the firepower, the driver performed a U-turn and sped to nearby Battersea Police Station where he ran inside. Detectives discovered he was wanted for questioning over a double killing at a party in north London on New Year's Day. The Wandsworth attack had been a contract revenge killing in which the only victim was an innocent man.

TRAFFICK ISLAND

According to Jamaican police there were around 500 known criminals from the island operating in Britain in 2002. The majority are affiliated to some 30 Yardie gangs — organizations with imaginative names such as the Kickoffhead Crew, the Lock City Crew, the Cartel Crew the African Crew, the British Link Up Crew, Clans Massive, the Black Roses and the President's Click. The Click was apparently formed out of the notorious Shower Posse gang, rumoured to have committed 1,400 murders in the USA.

Just like the New York and Chicago gangsters of the 1920s and 1930s the Jamaican networks began life as election 'muscle', bullies hired to ensure that voters would support either the left-wing People's National Party or the conservative Jamaican Labour Party. Whereas Al Capone and his Chicago associates got rich on bootlegged alcohol, the Yardie leaders realised that cocaine was their ticket to riches. On 10 February 2002 the London-based *Sunday Times* named the leader of the President's Click and quoted a Jamaican police officer as saying: 'He is wanted for everything – murder, drugs running, you name it. He is linked to gangs in the UK but he is untouchable because of his political links. That is the culture in Jamaica.'

A fortnight later, the same newspaper ran a two-page special quoting senior officers by name. Carl Williams, the superintendent in charge of the island's anti-narcotics squad, told reporters: 'People in Britain have an insatiable appetite for cocaine. We are providing them with it.'

Jamaican Special Branch superintendent Tony Hewitt agreed: 'It seems that every time you search for a man you hear that he is in England,' he said. 'They go all over your country. They are selling drugs in every city. It is not just London. Do you know, the last time I talked to a gunman I couldn't arrest he laughed and said: "A friend of mine has sent out a ticket from London and I'm going to go soon."'

DEALING WITH IT

British police have responded to the cocaine crimewave. Brown's Operation Trident arrested 441 people in 2001, most aged between 16 and 35. Of the 620 kilos of Class A drugs recovered nearly all was cocaine. Similar operations are ongoing: 'Stirrup', in Leeds, which resulted in 57 deportations to Jamaica in 2001; 'Atrium' in Bristol; 'Ventara' in Birmingham; 'Trojan' in Southampton; and 'Ovidian' in Plymouth.

Although Britain's crack market is Jamaican-controlled there is no evidence that the drug is used mostly in black communities. According to one senior Metropolitan Police detective it has penetrated all social backgrounds, with a 'heartland' of users – mostly beggars – in Soho, central London. This officer, a member of the London Crime Squad, heads an undercover team that buys crack on the street, busts key players and passes intelligence to other units. He has 21 years' experience, the past four in drugs operations.

'There is no great class divide,' he told me. 'Crack cocaine is used by all racial groups although beggars are the big market. If you go to black areas like Brixton you will obviously tend to find more black users. The same is true for white areas – particular in outer south-east London. There are several nightclubs where it is used by the black community but crack is not a club drug in the same league as, say, ecstasy.

'In areas of the West End, particularly around Soho, the customers are pretty much all vagrants. These are people who will beg for a quantity of pound coins until they have enough money to buy a stone. There is also a significant passing trade in office workers – men and women in suits – both black and white people.

'It's difficult to say whether crack actually turns people into beggars. People end up living on the streets for a variety of reasons and in central London you'll find a lot of young people, often children, who have run away from home. Inevitably they gravitate towards Soho, which is where the street dealers operate. If they experiment with crack and they get a habit then they pay for that habit through begging or crime.'

The Metropolitan Police anti-crack team pays maybe £20 (about $30) a stone (a piece of crack cocaine), which typically weighs about 200mg. Stones fluctuate from 50–60g (1¾–2oz) to around 300g (10½oz) and, like powder coke, they will have varying levels of purity depending on the recipe used to cook them. Maintaining a crack habit without a healthy income or resorting to prostitution is nigh on impossible, however good your sob story to passers-by.

'People talk glibly about smoking a dozen stones a day,' said the detective. 'That means the drug is costing them perhaps £200 ($290) daily and although there's a discount

Demand for help in beating cocaine abuse accounted for 30 per cent of all drug treatment admissions across 20 US cities during 1997. By contrast, demand in key European cities was just 3.5 per cent. Only Amsterdam (31 per cent) rivalled the US figure. UN office for Drug Control and Crime Prevention report, 2001

if they buy in bulk, crime is often the only way to pay. Users become desperate for crack and will do almost anything to get it. This may mean robbing someone in the street – especially if they need a stone urgently and haven't the means of finding money quickly. In the last four years crack crime has been a constant problem and it has escalated in that time.

'There's no such thing as a typical street dealer, but there are very few that have full-time jobs. We did find somebody who worked at a hairdresser's shop in the morning and then cruised the streets selling cocaine in the afternoon. Dealers basically work the hours they want to.

'Some sell straight to the crack houses. There are a plethora of these in London – addresses where users know they can go to smoke out of sight. It is a huge problem but it is almost impossible to estimate the total number of users. From our experience I would say the majority are aged under 30.'

He believes the fight against crack dealing is not hopeless, but demands a rolling review of police tactics. 'There is also an immigration issue here with carriers entering the UK, particularly from Jamaica,' he said. 'We need to look at these drug mules more closely and identify those who sponsor their application to enter Britain.'

Young, homeless, addicted, broke and desperate to service a craving for crack. No wonder cocaine has become synonymous with crime around the world. But if you think this is only a problem for the major cities think again. Crack dealers are businessmen. They thrive on making and defending new markets.

CRACK'S HOLIDAY HOME-FROM-HOME

The picturesque town of St Ives on the surf-battered north coast of Cornwall, England, has everything you'd expect from an unspoilt seaside resort. Rows of fishermen's cottages, narrow cobbled streets, wonderful fish restaurants, golden beaches, a world-renowned art gallery (the Tate) and boats bobbing at anchor in the sparkling waters of the harbour. St Ives also offers one thing you wouldn't expect from the Great British seaside experience. Of course, its not a blatant trade, but if you know where to go and who to ask, you can find plenty of rocks away from the beach.

The crack house could be anywhere. It will contain the usual unremarkable paraphernalia – glass jars and saucepans for cooking up, silver foil, weighing scales, dealers' client lists and plenty of ready cash. The crack will probably come in 200mg rocks, barely half the size of your fingernail. If you're buying on the street your dealer might carry the rock in his mouth, wrapped in clingfilm between his top lip and the gum. If there's a bust it's easier to swallow.

Before the outraged townsfolk of St Ives ceremoniously burn this book in the streets, let's get something clear. This is one small town among thousands worldwide where crack is available. It just illustrates the point that this drug is not confined to ghettos and run-down inner cities. Having picturesque streets and bucket-and-spade tourists around is not a huge deterrent to your average dealer.

Detective Sergeant Darren Lockley is part of the Devon and Cornwall police crime intelligence team that is hunting down crack dealers under Operation Ovidian. 'We know that this drug is already firmly rooted in the two counties and that established supply networks run to Bristol, London, Liverpool, Manchester and Birmingham,' he says. 'It is vitally important that everyone has an understanding about the use of crack cocaine and the violent culture surrounding it.

'The danger is complacency; believing that murders and drive-by shootings can't happen here. Other police forces that have thought this way are now suffering the consequences. We are trying to learn from their experience and prevent extreme violence on our patch.

'West Indian organized crime groups are extending the crack market right across the country. Political unrest in Jamaica is displacing top criminals to the UK. Dealers have already been flooding cities such as Bristol and London, and there have been some fairly brutal turf wars.

'Intelligence reports suggest that many users are spending £500 [$725] a day on their habit. In February 2002 we arrested one low-level supplier who was making £3,000 [$4,350] per day. We know this figure is accurate. We're talking about a supplier who was at the bottom of the chain and yet his income may have topped £1.2 million [$1.7 million] a year.'

Crack's combination of quick dependency, high availability and ease of preparation encourages addicts to commit street robberies to get instant cash. Typical users, said Lockley, need between £10,000 ($14,500) and £20,000 ($29,000) a year and in Plymouth, Devon (the focal point of the region's cocaine trade), crime figures have become distorted by the crack factor. In 2001 – the year Operation Ovidian was launched –

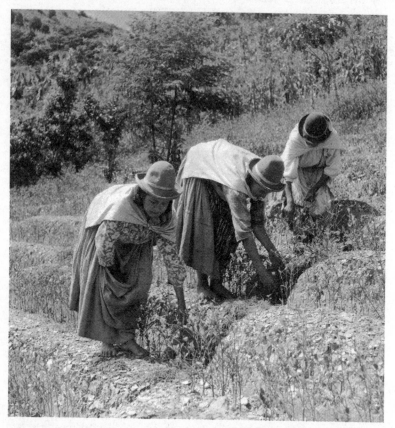

Women picking coca leaves during the harvest in the mountains near Chulumani, Bolivia. When the women tire, they chew leaves for stimulation.

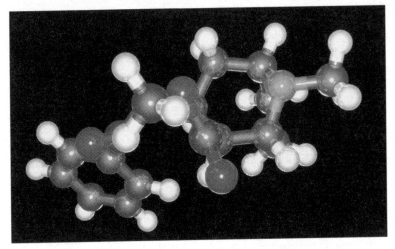

Molecular model of the drug cocaine (formula $C_{17}H_{21}NO_4$). As an alkaloid drug, cocaine has a powerful local anaesthetic action when applied to the skin and was often used in surgery. Due to its more notorious effects, however, it has largely been replaced by other anaesthetics.

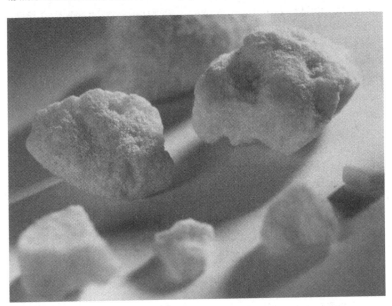

Rocks of crack cocaine. Crack is the street name for an almost pure form of cocaine. Conventional cocaine powder consists mostly of cocaine hydrochloride, which is destroyed by heating and therefore impossible to smoke, while crack is prepared by mixing ammonia with a solution of cocaine hydrochloride, which causes the alkaloidal pure cocaine to be precipitated. This is then compacted into 'rocks' and smoked in a pipe. The drug is absorbed through the lungs more quickly than snorted cocaine, producing an intense, extremely addictive, but short-lived rush.

the city saw a 12 per cent street crime increase, while other areas of Devon and Cornwall reported an average 6 per cent decrease for comparable offences.

'We know there is now an extremely viable crack market in Devon and Cornwall,' said Lockley. 'When we took out the dealer making £3,000 [$4,350] a day we arrested both him and the Jamaicans who were supplying him. Within a month the Jamaicans were replaced by other Jamaicans who immediately got other dealers in place. Despite the risk of arrest, the market is so valuable that it's worthwhile for them to bring more people in.

'They tend to target vulnerable people like prostitutes and heroin addicts. West Indian organized crime

> Of the 88,550 British offenders sentenced for using, possessing, dealing or trafficking illicit drugs in 1999, 4 per cent were involved with cocaine and 1 per cent with crack. The number of cocaine offences has risen steadily every year since 1994. The number of crack offences has risen more slowly but still almost doubled between 1996 and 1999.
> British Crime Survey, 2000

traditionally links up with prostitution for two reasons. One is that the gang leaders can easily bring prostitutes into the country and provide them with a safe house. They may even arrange marriage to allow the women to stay in the country longer.

'The other reason is that prostitutes are good at networking within the criminal fraternity. They can help identify potential new dealers who will be introduced to crack through special offers, say a large rock for the price of a small one. It's a market just like any other but it uses extreme levels of violence to maintain control.

'There's evidence that Jamaican crack suppliers are also bringing in heroin because they know that a lot of users will binge on crack and then use heroin to manage the come-down. It brings the Jamaican gangs into conflict with established heroin suppliers and that means a turf war. Operators start "taxing" each other – robbing their rivals' supplies.

'A dealer will order crack from his supplier and then sell it to users at a pre-arranged time and place. We had one incident in February [2002] in which a Jamaican dealer was confronted by three others from a rival gang who were going to tax him. During the taxing he received an ice pick in his head and was stabbed. We thought we were looking at murder but amazingly the guy came through.

'There's also a public order issue. In 2002 there was fighting on the streets of Plymouth to get to one particular dealer – simply because demand was so great. You've got people waiting to meet their man and there's a fight in the queue because someone can't wait any longer. This is the problem with crack. Users forget everything – the law, social niceties, their own values. One of them described it to us as comparable to an all-over body orgasm. They care only about getting the drug.

'Cocaine is worth three times more in this country than it is in Jamaica, which is why so much of it comes here. But if you turn it into crack you will always make more money than from powder. You know your customers will always want you and because of the greater purity and intense high you can charge what the market will stand. What police have found in Bristol is that you don't get many powder cocaine seizures now – it's mostly just crack.

'We've got crack in every corner of our region – Penzance, Ilfracombe, St Ives. If you've ever been to St Ives you'll know it's a beautiful place. Unfortunately beautiful places won't escape crack cocaine.'

WHAT'S THE SET-UP?
Street dealers use a variety of business models. The most basic has a single trader buying and selling small quantities, often to fund his own habit. More usually (according to Pearson and Hobbs) there will be a team centred on a leader who buys wholesale and assigns runners to make street deliveries or take payments. This leader maintains the books and keeps the contacts hot. There may also be peripheral employees, eg purity testers, crack cooks and packagers.

Results of the UK Home Office's New English and Welsh Arrestee Drug Abuse Monitoring programme (NEW-ADAM), published in 2000, looked at cocaine and crack purchases in two British cities: Nottingham and Sunderland. Of the 131-strong sample, 82 per cent bought in their local neighbourhood and 75 per cent made contact with their dealer via a pager or mobile phone.

Two-thirds were given a collection point (usually in a residential street) while the remainder had it delivered to their door by a courier.

In America cocaine markets traditionally work on a credit system in which the drug is supplied up-front by wholesalers to street dealers. The dealer than pays up over an agreed timescale. In the UK this model is less typical; sometimes cash on delivery is demanded within a network and sometimes it isn't. Either way it makes sense to keep drug and cash runners separate. If there's a bust or a taxing it means there's less to lose.

London's Metropolitan Police Force is resorting to increasingly sneaky tactics to raid cocaine dealers. On Saturday 23 March 2002, dozens of officers arrived outside a pub in Edgware, north London, in a double-decker bus to ensure they were less conspicuous. Ten people were arrested and cocaine and weapons seized.

Dealers who peddle only one type of drug are comparatively rare. Marijuana is an exception because it is seen as all but legal. Why would grass-only suppliers wish to jeopardize a good business by dabbling in a drug like coke, with all the additional hassle from police and rival operators that might bring? Often street dealers will buy from 'multi-commodity brokers' offering club drugs such as speed, ecstasy, powder coke and perhaps a little marijuana on the side. Finally, there is the crack and heroin market, seen as a class apart because it involves 'dirty' habits. Even dealers and traffickers have morals ...

... but not all of them. The level of violence used to extract payments and warn off competitors has no comparison in the criminal underworld. This occurs mostly at international trafficking level (see the section on Colombian drug barons in Chapter 3), but sometimes also between rival gangs in an individual city. None of the players goes looking for trouble because it stirs up police interest and is generally bad for business. Usually it's the sign of an unstable, disrupted supply chain or a good old-fashioned turf war.

NECESSARY VIOLENCE?
Kidnapping has been a speciality of the Colombian cocaine rings. Say a Colombian distributor living in London reneges on a deal. He may find that

his mother or sister back home is abducted and held until the debt is paid. At a lower level, dealers have been known to lose expensive cars – held as surety until they settle their dues. Overt physical violence is often a last resort but Pearson and Hobbs quote one example in which enforcers from a middle-market broker met a debtor at a country pub. Despite offering to pay he was taken hostage and severely beaten until both his hands were broken. He was later found naked and badly injured, rolled up in a carpet behind a fish-and-chip shop.

Another, more disturbing, example involved a small-time loner who owed comparatively little in drug debts. Because he had no back-up of his own it was convenient to humiliate and torture him as an example to other bad payers.

'He was beaten on the arms and legs with iron bars, made to dress in women's clothes and apply lipstick to himself and various objects were inserted into his anus. Photographs were taken of his humiliating circumstances and then shown around to local people with a clear message: "This is what happens if you mess with us"' (Pearson and Hobbs).

However, not all cocaine dealers see violence as necessary. One 31-year-old British male prisoner who bought cocaine in kilo loads and distributed it by the ounce (28g) saw it as pointless and self-defeating.

'All we used to say was "Listen, here's what. You let me down then you don't get it again." Simple as that. Don't even come knocking on the door. But none of this "I'll threaten to do this or that" ... that's what makes people more on edge, and if they're on edge they can do silly things. They always say don't be scared of the hard man, be scared of the frightened man' (Pearson and Hobbs).

Another British male prisoner, aged 34, agreed. 'So a guy owes me a grand,' he said. 'I can turn that around in a day, no sweat, in a few hours. Why go hunting the mug down to give him a good hiding. Wasting time. Time's money. Just get back to work making money' (Pearson and Hobbs).

> '*It was the height of hedonism; drug-taking and four-in-a-bed sex, sometimes homosexual and sometimes heterosexual. I don't suppose their partners ever knew what was going on.*'
>
> – Customs source on the lifestyle of two drug traffickers

COKE AT WORK AND PLAY

To appreciate the forces that drive worldwide cocaine trafficking you first have to crunch statistics. Drugs breed statistics. So this next bit is for all those anoraks who feel comfortable knowing that in Guatemala the annual prevalence of cocaine abuse as a percentage of the population aged 15 or over in 1998 was 1.6 per cent (*Global Illicit Drug Trends*, United Nations, 2001).

The Vienna-based United Nations International Drug Control Programme is a mine of fascinating facts on cocaine. In 2001 it estimated that the drug was used by 0.3 per cent of the global population with more than 70 per cent of these consumers living in North or South America and 16 per cent in Europe. Abuse levels in North America were seven times the world average, while Asians and eastern Europeans were noticeably abstemious. The continental breakdown is shown in the table below.

NUMBER OF COCAINE USERS (MILLIONS) AS A PERCENTAGE OF POPULATION AGED 15+

	MILLIONS	% OF POPULATION AGED 15+
North America	7.0	2.20
South America	3.1	1.10
Oceania	0.2	0.90
Western Europe	2.2	0.70
Eastern Europe	0.1	0.04
Africa	1.3	0.30
Asia	0.2	0.01
Global	14	0.30

WORLD OF COCAINE

More important than the hard data is the trend in consumption levels. Here's what the UNDCP's *Global Illicit Drug Trends* (GIDT) report for 2001 has to say about the pattern of cocaine use around the world. Most of the statistics are two to three years old (it takes this long to collect, collate and publish them) and there is inevitably a variation in sampling methods.

THE AMERICAS

Annual cocaine use (ie taking at least once a year) has stabilized in North America at 1.7 per cent of the population aged 12 and above. This is one-third lower than in 1985, while the number of monthly users fell even more dramatically over the same timespan – from 3 per cent to 0.7 per cent.

One illuminating section of the GIDT report is the 'Use, Risk, Disapproval and Availability' survey 2000, which looks at attitudes to cocaine and crack among American schoolchildren. This showed that just over 4 per cent of twelfth-graders used cocaine powder (down from 10 per cent in 1987). Half of the sample group said they saw 'great risk' in using it once or twice (same as 1987), 85 per cent said they disapproved of using once or twice (same as 1987) and just over 40 per cent said it was easy to get hold of (down from 50 per cent in 1987).

For crack, the figures revealed that 2 per cent of twelfth-graders in the sample had used in the past year (half the 1987 figure). Just under 50 per cent thought there were great risks attached to occasional use (down from 60 per cent in 1987). Around 85 per cent disapproved of using once or twice (slight decline on 1987) and 40 per cent said it was easy to obtain (same as 1987).

On the whole, these figures look encouraging for the US government. However the report points out that even with a projected decline to 5.5 million users by 2000, the USA will remain far and away the world's biggest coke market.

Elsewhere in the Americas cocaine use is mostly on the increase. Peru and Bolivia – the two biggest coca leaf producers – are notable exceptions. Surveys there show a decline in the number of people experimenting with the drug during the 1990s. Brazil, Argentina and Chile now have the highest percentage of 'lifetime prevalence' cocaine powder abusers outside the USA. In Argentina the percentage of annual users is 1.9 per cent and in Chile 1.3 per cent. Colombia – the 'home of cocaine' – appears to have stable abuse levels (1.6 per cent of the population are lifetime users), although this figure was recorded back in 1996.

EUROPE
Data shows that Europe's two biggest cocaine markets – the UK and Spain – have stabilized. In contrast there is increasing use in Germany, France, The Netherlands, Belgium, Denmark, Norway, Portugal, Cyprus and Turkey. Eastern European countries barely perceive it as a problem. 'Cocaine in Europe – similar to the USA in the 1970s prior to the crack epidemic – is often used recreationally and constitutes less of a social problem than in North America,' says the report.

'However, there has been a trend towards poly-drug abuse ... many heroin addicts consume cocaine, increasingly in the form of crack. Similarly, there have been reports across western Europe of people on methadone maintenance programmes using cocaine to get their "kick".'

Another insight comes from the Brussels liaison department of the United Nations Office of Drug Control and Crime Prevention (UNODCCP). In 2001 it was generally upbeat about the trend in Europe. 'There was an increase in cocaine trafficking and consumption in Europe over the last decade – and this upward trend is probably going to continue. But it has been a creeping increase and there are no indications that this trend is likely to change dramatically in the near future. There are reports of youths who used to take ecstasy changing over to cocaine and there are reports of cocaine spreading from the upper class (or upper middle class) to other sections of society. But all of these trends do not appear – at least for the time being – to result in what could be called a cocaine epidemic.'

The UNODCCP also points out how the political history of a country can significantly affect consumption. In western Germany the number of people taking cocaine at least annually amounted to 0.7 per cent of the population in 1997, whereas in the eastern part of the country, the 'closed' provinces formerly under a communist regime reported a total of just

0.1 per cent. Presumably the Berlin Wall was a bummer for traffickers. Similarly, 'Only Spain, which has traditionally close links with its former colonies in Latin America, including the Andean region, has abuse levels of cocaine which approach those of the USA.' Spain's annual prevalence figure in 1997 was 1.5 per cent of the 15–65 age group.

The UNODCCP report concludes that 'Cocaine use in Europe is already widespread among people in entertainment, in the media and communications and some groups of professionals. There are no indications that the spread of cocaine among these sections of society is on the rise – they are rather ageing while using cocaine. Social security institutions may have to pay in one way or another for the resulting health problems. But use within these circles does not necessarily lead to a spread as members – usually – do not make their living out of drug trafficking.

'If there is an increase in cocaine use it could be expected to arise primarily among ageing groups of the "ecstasy generation" who may try to experiment with other drugs as well, including cocaine. But these groups – though representing potential health problem for themselves and for society at large – are at least less prone to undergo cocaine-related criminal activities than deprived youths living in some ghettos.'

> In the United States, wholesale cocaine prices ranged from $12,000 (£8,300) to $35,000 (£24,000) per kilo (2¼lb) during 2000. In urban areas the spread was much narrower: $13,000 (£9,000) to $25,000 (£17,250). Seizures showed an average purity level of 75 per cent. *Drug Trafficking In The United States*, Drug Enforcement Administration, September 2001

AFRICA AND ASIA

The GIDT report reveals that cocaine abuse is largely a southern and western Africa phenomena. From the figures available there is increasing use in the Republic of South Africa and, especially, Angola (reflecting trafficking links with Brazil). Most cocaine shipped to Africa is intended for a final destination in Europe. Asian governments regard cocaine as a low-priority social issue. In 1999 only seven countries bothered to report trends in consumption and most of these were stable or falling.

OCEANIA
Australia is facing one of the biggest rises in cocaine abuse. The number of annual users almost tripled between 1993 and 1998 (from 0.5 per cent to 1.4 per cent of the population aged 14 and above), equivalent to the highest national rates found in Europe. This trend has not permeated to New Zealand, where year-on-year consumption is said to be stable.

PURER EQUALS MORE
One good indicator of coke availability can be found in the purity of police seizures. According to the 2001 GIDT report, 'As prices tend to remain rather stable in the drug markets, short-term changes in supply are usually reflected in shifts in purities. Higher levels of purities indicate improved supply.' In other words a street dealer with loads of Charlie on his hands doesn't worry too much about cutting. He passes on the improved quality to his buyers – just like any other customer-focused business.

The UNODCCP says that in 1999, mean cocaine purities exceeded 62 per cent in Britain. The last time purity levels topped this benchmark was in 1989 (it has ranged between 47 per cent and 55 per cent throughout the decade). While prosecution and seizure statistics will highlight bits of the story, most analysts agree that there's nothing like good old market forces to get to the nub of things. Cocaine powder 62 per cent pure is not a resounding victory for the forces of British law and order, and is a statistically significant change for the worse ... or better, depending on your point of view.

To put the problem into some kind of perspective, let's take a look at the comments of Britain's deputy high commissioner to Jamaica, Phil Sinkinson. On 2 January 2002 he was asked by BBC Radio 4's *Today* programme to comment on newspaper claims that one in every ten air passengers travelling from Jamaica to Britain was a cocaine carrier or 'drug mule'. His response? 'Probably an estimate on the low side.'

By the spring of 2002 there were 14 flights a week from Jamaica into London's Gatwick and Heathrow airports. Given that these aircraft carry an average of 237 passengers per flight, and that at least a tenth of all passengers are said to be smuggling half a kilo (1lb) of cocaine apiece (a conservative guess), the combined weekly haul is 166kg (365lb). After cutting with glucose, lactose, Novocain or, on a bad day, scouring powder, the imported weight would increase by maybe a third. The sums then add up like this: 220kg (485lb) of cut powder x £63,000 ($91,000) (the average street price per kilo/2¼lb) = £13.8 million ($20 million). Remember this is one week, two airports and a few cautious estimates. Why would anyone want to work for a living?

Falling street prices are another general indicator of oversupply. Powder coke prices have generally been dropping worldwide throughout the last decade despite steadily rising numbers of seizures by police and customs. In America, prices halved between 1996 and 1999 to around $30 (£20) per gram despite the number of seizures increasing from 54,881kg (50 tons) to 84,700kg (76 tons) over the same period (according to the United States' Drug Enforcement Administration).

In Britain, there was an 18 per cent average price fall in 1999 alone – down from £77 ($112) to £63 ($91) per gram. The UNODCCP breezily notes that 'though cocaine prices still vary significantly from country to country, data also show that price discrepancies are becoming less pronounced, reflecting a European unification process that also affects the cocaine market.'

While the number of users has stabilized in America this should not be confused with the level of consumption. In the USA, the number of coke-related hospital emergency room incidents doubled from 80,355 in 1990 to 161,087 in 1997, indicating that Uncle Sam has been harbouring some fairly heavy snorters'n'smokers. This ER figure has since come down. In Europe, Spain leads the league table of cocaine consumption (just 20 per cent lower than the USA) followed by the UK, The Netherlands and Germany.

GERMANY

Ah yes, Germany. The nation that first produced cocaine back in the 19th century (see Chapter 3) has never quite ended its love affair with the drug. During the 1990s the decline in its street cocaine price was greater than anywhere else in Europe – it fell by two-thirds between 1996 and 1998. At Europe's busiest air hub, Frankfurt Airport, customs officers seized 780kg (1,720lbs) of the drug in 1995, compared to 421kg (925lbs) the previous year.

In the first six months of 1999, according to the UNODCCP, 45 per cent of all cocaine seized in Germany was in transit to other European countries.

In fact, the 1997 report of Geopolitical Drug Watch (you're right, it could only be funded by the European Commission) revealed that cocaine dealing in Germany 'has broken out of its closed circle of distributors and consumers and has taken on the same mass character as heroin dealing. Those arrested include Nigerians, Italians, South Americans and Eastern European nationals, but most were Germans; this diversity clearly demonstrates the splintering and democratization of the market.'

Democracy and cocaine is something the Bundestag knows all about. In October 2000 an undercover TV reporter strolled around Germany's parliament building visiting 28 men's toilets and wiping down their surfaces with paper tissues. The tissues were stuffed into airtight tubes and analysed by the Nuremberg-based forensic analyst Professor Fritz Sorgel. He found that 22 out of the 28 carried traces of cocaine.

Sorgel stressed that his findings might have been distorted by cleaners spreading the drug around on their cloths. Others were less restrained. 'The Parliament of Addicts', declared the tabloid paper *BZ*. Hubert Huppe, the Christian Social Union's narcotics spokesman, pointed out that 'it would be unnatural if parliamentarians were the only group to have nothing to do with drugs'.

There's no question that Germans enjoy a bit of substance abuse. They smoke and drink more than most Europeans and it's thought that more than half a million of them take cocaine every year. Two-thirds of these users dabble more than once a month and 75,000 have a daily habit. Unless they're suspected of dealing, these people have nothing to fear from the police because taking drugs is not punishable by law.

The Bundestag bog-snorting scandal provoked a flurry of stories about Berlin coke-heads at play. The best concerned a restaurant party thrown a few months earlier by a fashion designer who sent aides scurrying off to complain that the toilet extractor fans were too powerful. No one could lay out a line because cocaine was blowing everywhere.

Then there was the incident reported in *Der Spiegel* (October 2000) recounting a reading in a trendy Berlin cabaret theatre. The writer of the work sat in the front row helping himself to liberal quantities of coke from an envelope. In the bar later he formed lines into the shape of a swastika and urged friends to snort them. There was only one complaint and that was from a woman who claimed the commotion had delayed her getting served.

THE BUSINESS

One explanation of cocaine's tacit acceptance among Germany's middle classes is that employers may not necessarily see it as a Bad Thing. At the height of the Bundestag business a leading social scientist, Gunter Amendt, pointed out that whereas marijuana and alcohol were 'employer unfriendly', the big C actually makes staff graft harder. There's nothing new about this idea – for centuries South American plantation owners even paid their workforce with it – but in a nation with Germany's enhanced work ethic you can see how it might appeal.

'The constant, excessive demands made on our imagination, our emotions and our responsibility has increased demand for pharmacological aids to restore a balanced personality,' said Amendt. This conjures up wonderful images of future industrial relations. Imagine BMW's production figures with the night shift on coke rations. If this sounds like something from an Aldous Huxley novel remember that on Wall Street allegations have been flying about employers who condone cocaine use among staff.

One woman who ran a small brokerage trading desk with her husband claimed his $500-a-day (£350) habit was happily tolerated by his bosses. They realised it was good for business as some clients liked to take 'sweeteners' in powder form. And we're not talking about that other well-known synthetic, white crystalline substance known as saccharin.

> Ships used to smuggle cocaine into the United States are treated in uncompromising fashion. On 6 June 2001 the US Customs Service announced plans to 'deep six' (ie sink) three cargo ships off the coast of Miami to create an artificial reef and marine wildlife habitat.

Research aimed specifically at 'non-deviants' (that's social science speak for anyone who's not a criminal, a prostitute or an addict under treatment) re-affirms cocaine's social kudos. A study of 268 regular users by Peter Cohen and Arjan Sas (*Cocaine Use In Amsterdam In Non Deviant Subcultures*, 1994) showed that 75 per cent came from good high school or university backgrounds, 84 per cent were aged between 20 and 35, and 60 per cent were in full or part-time employment.

While occupations were varied, large subgroups included students (15 per cent), art and art-related careers (24 per cent), professionals such as doctors, managers, high-level administrators and teachers (15 per cent), and 'medium strata' employees such as nurses and hairdressers (20 per cent). Cohen and Sas suggested that a cocaine habit did not necessarily disrupt working lives and that self-regulation rather than law enforcement was the main preventative factor. 'Extended careers of cocaine use, lasting even a decade, do not inevitably culminate in compulsive and/or destructive use or "addiction",' they concluded.

HARD TO HANDLE?

This is the abiding mystery of cocaine culture. How come some take it without a problem while others watch their personal lives and careers mercilessly shredded? One of the most brilliant economists on Wall Street, Lawrence Kudlow, was earning $1 million (£700,000) a year when he started snorting as a 25 year old in 1984. As an adviser to the Reagan administration he was courted and cosseted by the markets to the point that he felt 'indestructible'. Then he began missing client appointments and got himself fired from the investment bank Bear Stearns. The cocaine vice gripped ever stronger; debts mounted; his wife threatened divorce.

In 1995, Kudlow went into five months of rehab. He kicked his addiction, became a devout Christian and, in 2000, regained the giddy heights of Wall Street as chief economist to ING Barings. 'Handling large sums of money can sometimes mislead people into thinking that they are powerful,' he said in one interview in November 2000. 'They are not. I have never blamed Wall Street. It's an attitude, not the pressure. People believe they can turn it on and turn it off and, sooner or later, they realise that they can't.'

Manhattan-based addiction therapist Dr Arnold Washton, founder of America's first cocaine hotline in 1982, sees this all the time. Around a third of his clients work on Wall Street and they tell him they use the drug to feel 'energetic, powerful, sexy and on top of the world'. Washton has little doubt that cocaine is re-emerging as the drug of choice for senior executives. 'It was almost treated as passé for a while,' he told the London *Guardian* (29 November 2000). 'There's a new crop of young, ambitious professionals who find this drug suitable. It fits right in with the tenor of the times.'

It is exactly this attitude that so angers some senior politicians and police officers. On 4 January 1999, Britain's so-called 'drugs tsar', Keith Hellawell, waded into City of London cocaine users. Just because wealth allowed them to buy the drug without thieving, he told BBC Radio 4's *Today* programme, it didn't mean they were innocent of damaging society. 'I wish they'd stop it,' he said. 'There's this arrogance – I call it an intellectual arrogance. If they are dealing with my pension fund on the dealing floors they could be causing me damage. It isn't a joke, it's deadly serious.'

SPORTING SNORTERS

This is another strange facet of the cocaine debate. Sometimes it's funny, sometimes it's not. When the England international footballer Robbie Fowler celebrated a goal at his former club Liverpool FC by kneeling down and running his nose along the white line of the penalty area, everybody under 40 in the crowd had a good laugh. This generation was familiar with cocaine; they knew Fowler was comparing the 'high' of scoring with the 'high' of coke.

Yet for those world-famous sportsmen and women caught using the drug the consequences are stark. When Germany appointed Christoph Daum as trainer of its national football team in 2000 there were widespread rumours that his trademark 'boggle-eyed' expression and legendary short temper were the result of cocaine use. Daum agreed to have a hair sample analysed to prove his innocence. It was the worst result of his career. The test showed he'd consumed large quantities of the drug and the coaching offer was hurriedly withdrawn.

Drug testing has now become so prevalent in sport that for professional players and athletes a line or two of cocaine is no longer worth the risk. American footballer Dexter Manley failed one test while starring for the

Washington Redskins in 1989 and then another two years later as a Tampa Bay Buccaneers player. He retired from football but not from cocaine and eventually served 15 months of a four-year drugs sentence.

In March 2002 he was again jailed by a court in Houston, Texas, after a jury found that he'd tried to swallow less than a gram during a drug bust at a city motel. The judge told him he needed mental health counselling because he'd become so self-destructive. 'I did it to myself,' Manley told TV crews as he was hustled away to start a two-year stretch. 'I apologize to the fans and public.' This is not quite true. He needed a little help from his friends in Central and South America. He couldn't have done it without the traffickers.

> In the first seven months of 2001 Spanish anti-drug agencies seized a total of 25 tonnes/tons of cocaine from areas as diverse as the northern Basque region, the Mediterranean coast and the waters off French Guyana in the Caribbean. If this had been cut and laid out as a continuous 'line' it would have stretched for 12,500km (7,500 miles).
> BBC News, 19 August 2001

FREE-FLOWING TRAFFIC

Cocaine consumers may come from all walks of life but the cocaine business has only one spiritual home. It's true that Peru is probably the largest coca leaf grower, that Bolivia harvests a decent crop, that Mexican drug cartels have grabbed a big slice of the US smuggling trade, and that the Caribbean is a key worldwide transiting centre. There are growers and traffickers in Brazil, Venezuela, Argentina, Ecuador, Uruguay and Paraguay, but you could take down every last one and barely register a blip on world supplies. There is only one undisputed king of the cocaine ring. Ask any law enforcement agency and they'll tell you: 80 per cent of the world's cocaine moves through Colombia.

According to the UN special conference on the global drug problem (New York, 1998) there has been a big reduction in area devoted to the coca bush worldwide. In 1990 this stood at 288,000ha (710,000 acres); by 1998 it was down to 179,000ha (440,000 acres). Yet the production of coca in tonnes has seen a more gradual decline – from 363,981 tonnes/tons in 1990 to around 300,000 in 1998. A combination of improving crop yields (horticultural science doesn't care who it helps) and the spread of new, unidentified plantations probably explains the discrepancy.

Despite a 40 per cent reduction in its coca crop, Peru is theoretically the biggest grower (118,000 tonnes/tons in 1997) followed by Bolivia (93,000 tonnes/tons) and Colombia (91,000 tonnes/tons). By the time this book is published this league table may well have changed as Colombian guerrillas use coca growing to fund their continuing civil war against the government. What these statistics don't reveal is the proportion of South American coca bought up by Colombians. Put it this way, they don't miss much.

Assuming a conversion rate in which 1,000 tonnes/tons of coca leaf equals 9 tonnes/tons of cocaine, the UN reckons that the total world harvest was upwards of 800 tonnes/tons in 1997. Government seizures accounted for perhaps 300 tonnes/tons, leaving 500–700 tonnes/tons to be smuggled, shuffled, smoked and snorted around the globe. This is almost certainly a massive underestimate but then that's the United Nations for you.

The UN's *Global Illicit Drug Trends* report for 2001 has cast a little more light on things. It analyzed the amount of cocaine actually seized by government forces in 1999. This predictably showed the world's biggest market – America – way out in front with 132,318kg (291,000lbs). Next came Colombia with 63,945kg (140,000lbs) and way behind in third place Mexico with 34,623kg (76,000lbs).

The rest are also-rans. There's Spain (18,111kg/40,000lbs) Venezuela, Peru, The Netherlands, Ecuador and Guatemala (all in the 10,000–12,500kg/22,000–27,500lbs range) and Bolivia and Brazil (each 7,700kg/17,000lbs). The whole of western Europe accounted for 43,707kg (96,000lbs) while in the Caribbean, seizures amounted to 12,133kg (26,700lbs).

The report confirmed what everyone already knew: that the main trafficking routes shoot out from the major South and Central American producers and head straight up Uncle Sam's monster pair of nostrils in the north. Cocaine shipments come via road across the US/Mexican border, in 'go-fast' boats up America's Pacific coast and in sea ferries, pleasure boats or commercial planes via the Bahamas, Haiti, Puerto Rico, the Dominican Republic and various other Caribbean islands.

Jamaica is the main air bridge for Colombian cartels accessing Europe and the Middle East. Since the late 1990s these markets have been particularly good at filling traffickers' boots with cash, at only slightly enhanced levels of risk. Whereas a kilo (2¼lbs) of pure cocaine may sell for $20,000 (£14,000) wholesale in Miami, in London it can be worth three times as much. Elsewhere there is some traditional, international trade – Brazil to Angola, Ecuador to Hong Kong or Japan and Argentina to South Africa and Australia. As for smuggling methods, these range from the ingenious to the downright yucky (see below).

WHAT'S ON THE MOVE?

At this point we need to be clear about the type of cocaine being smuggled. If it's a bulk shipment it may be coca paste – *pasta basica* – the same, smokeable stuff that so excited those early American traffickers back in the 1970s and later sparked the crack epidemic. If it has already been fully processed it'll be pure(ish) cocaine hydrochloride in ready-to-cut powder form.

Paste is favoured by the big cocaine cartels because it's convenient in size and weight, and dead simple to produce in jungle kitchens from raw coca. The recipe varies from country to country, but essentially you harvest your coca leaves, dry them, chop them up, sprinkle them with cement and soak them in petrol for a day. This leaches out the cocaine alkaloid. You then siphon off the petrol and put the mashed leaves through a press to extract the remaining liquid.

Add a bucket of water containing some drops of car battery acid (one bucket per 30kg/65lbs of leaf), stir and allow to rest. Because the alkaloid is more soluble in acid than in petrol it moves into the acid solution. Chuck in some caustic soda, filter the solidifying murky mess through a cloth, strain and allow to dry into a yellowy-white powder. Here's your paste, somewhere between 40 and 60 per cent pure. If anyone ever tells you that cocaine is a 'natural' drug, ask them about the cement, petrol, battery acid and caustic soda. Jeez, no wonder your nose can rot.

In fairness, there are two further steps before the cocaine is ready for market. It has to be dissolved in solvents, allowed to solidify and then washed in another, very pure, solvent to produce 90 per cent pure cocaine

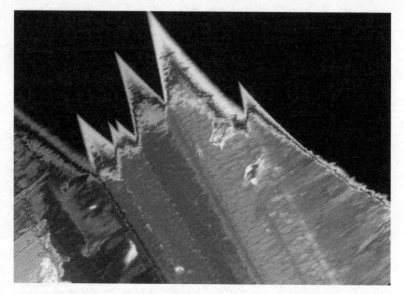

Polarised-light micrograph of crack cocaine crystals.

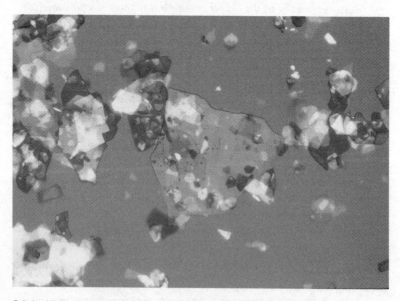

Polarised-light micrograph of crystals of pure, pharmaceutical-grade cocaine.

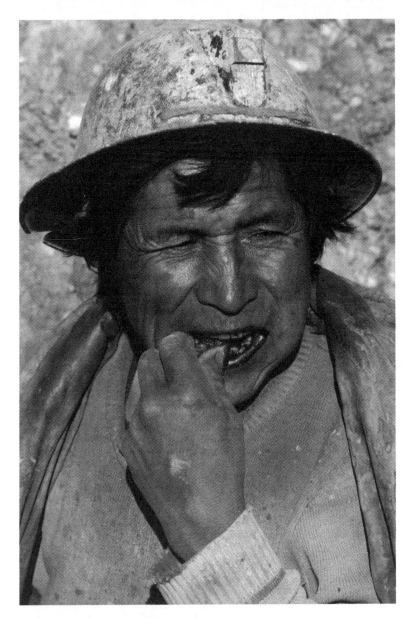

Bolivian miner chewing coca leaves, pressing a wad of dried leaves against his cheek. The narcotic principle is the alkaloid cocaine, of which the leaves contain about 1 per cent. It acts directly on the central nervous system, causing psychic exaltation and resistance to physical and mental fatigue. The use of coca leaves as a stimulating masticatory has been widespread among the people of the Amazon basin for many centuries. Cultivation was even encouraged by Jesuit missionaries.

hydrochloride. This is usually done by the cartel buyers, who process the paste in their own remote laboratories. It's at this point that the traffickers, and the money movers, queue up to make their millions.

WHO ARE THE MOVERS?

In September 2001 the US Office of Domestic Intelligence (ODI) published a report highlighting recent trends in the Central American cocaine markets. This showed that while Colombia remains the major player, drug cartels there have contracted-out much of their cross-border smuggling business to the Mexicans. Until 1989 Colombians usually paid Mexican traffickers to drive or fly cocaine across the US border (65 per cent of American cocaine enters this way) but had associates in place the other side to take delivery. This ensured that Colombian cartels retained control of wholesale distribution. However a massive 21 tonne/ton seizure in 1989 led to a new underworld deal.

'By the mid-1990s, Mexico-based transportation groups were receiving up to half the cocaine shipment they smuggled for the Colombia-based groups in exchange for their services,' says the ODI. 'Both sides realised that this strategy eliminated the vulnerabilities and complex logistics associated with large cash transactions. The Colombia-based groups also realised that relinquishing part of each cocaine shipment to their associates operating from Mexico ceded a share of the wholesale cocaine market in the United States.'

According to the ODI there then followed a good old-fashioned carve-up of territory. The Colombians retained control of their lucrative north-east markets and eastern seaboard cities such as Boston, Miami, Newark, New York and

Britain's greatest cocaine 'supergrass' is Michael Michael, caught running a £49 million ($71 million) trafficking operation centred on a coach nicknamed the 'Fun Bus'. Michael's plea bargaining led to 34 of his accomplices being jailed for more than 170 years. He escaped with a six-year sentence and will be given a new identity when he is freed. *Guardian* court report, 19 December 2001

Philadelphia. The Mexicans got the west and mid-west, specifically cities such as Chicago, Dallas, Denver, Houston, Los Angeles, Phoenix, San Diego, San Francisco and Seattle. Both sides made alliances with Dominican underworld groups (traditionally responsible for street-level distribution), particularly in New York City.

It's not that Colombian drug lords didn't have the stomach for a turf war. It's just that they didn't see the point. When you make $10 million (£7 million) a day, why worry if it drops to $5 million (£3.5 million), especially if the risks are spread. More to the point, there was that horrible word 'extradition', which had never really been part of the Colombian vocabulary. From 17 December 1997, however, any Colombian mafia boss drug-running overtly to the USA knew it was likely to lead to an appointment with an American judge. And a long, long time to think about what went wrong.

Incidentally, want to know what a Colombian mafia boss looks like? No problem. Log on to the Drug Enforcement Administration's website (any search engine will find it) and click on 'traffickers'. You'll get a neat passport-size picture of the people the DEA would dearly love to meet, together with their names and a short biography of the allegations against them. American law being what it is, you can accuse anyone of anything – even after you've arrested them – and still not prejudice a fair trial.

There's not much point in naming names here because, well, a week is a long time in the cocaine business. Even the most powerful figures in Colombia and Mexico have to watch their backs for a drive-by assassination or police shoot-out. In February 2002 I checked the DEA's website file on a notorious Mexican drugs baron called Ramon Arellano-Felix, one of three brothers running a 'powerful, violent and aggressive' trafficking group.

Ramon is identified as chief security honcho and most violent of the three. Not any more. Two weeks later I picked up the London *Observer* newspaper to learn that he'd been blown away by police gunmen. His battered Volkswagen had failed to stop at a routine check-point in the Pacific beach resort of Mazatlan, Mexico. You see the problem.

The Arellano-Felix Organization (AFO) was the cartel model used for Steven Soderbergh's award-winning film *Traffic* (still the best fictional portrayal of the cocaine business). This is the same Tijuana-based organization rumoured to spend $75 million (£50 million) a year bribing government officials. Since 1996, at least six Mexican generals have been imprisoned over links to the cartel – and that included the head of the army's anti-drug operations. It routinely murders police commanders, judges, politicians and lawyers – sometimes rousing them and their families from bed to parade in front of a machine-pistol firing squad.

In one 1996 killing the AFO shot a state prosecutor more than 100 times before disfiguring his body by repeatedly driving a van over it. It is also suspected of killing a three-year-old boy, gutting him and stuffing his body with cocaine. The body was strapped into a child seat and driven across the US/Mexican border. The *Observer* report (10 March 2002) adds, 'Fearless and supremely confident, Ramon once tested a new gun by simply shooting the first person he passed in his car, confident that no one in his home town would dare report the crime.'

Since Ramon's death, though, things have not gone well for the AFO, or indeed the Mexican underworld in general. On 9 March 2002, another Arellano-Felix brother, Benjamin, was arrested by Mexican police in Puebla. Then, on 28 March, a top lieutenant in the Gulf cartel, Adan Medrano Rodriguez, was captured in Mexico City. He had made the serious mistake of threatening two FBI agents in the border town of Matamoros in November 1999, whereupon the USA immediately offered a $2 million (£1.4 million) reward for information on his whereabouts.

Others facing charges in 2002 include Miguel Caro Quintero, head of the Sonora cartel, and a former Mexican state governor, Mario Villanueva, accused of helping to smuggle 200 tonnes/tons of cocaine to the USA on behalf of the Juarez cartel. This string of successes has given Mexican President Vicente Fox's government new clout in its dealings with the Bush administration.

It took Mexican police four weeks to realise that they had killed Ramon Arellano-Felix. Soon after the shooting some people arrived claiming to be family members, took away the body and had it cremated. FBI file pictures were of little help – they showed Ramon with a chubby face and facial features very different to those of the deceased. Eventually DNA tests on blood recovered from the scene settled the riddle. It was Ramon. He'd just had a little plastic surgery.

When a Colombian or Mexican drug lord dies accidentally or through natural causes no one ever believes it. People just assume the man concerned has faked his own death in order to acquire a clean new identity.

This is why good plastic surgeons are never idle in Central America. However, treating mafia bosses is not without the occasional setback, chief among which is the patient dying on the operating table. Drug families are never very understanding about that sort of thing.

So when Amado Carrillo Fuentes — the single most powerful cocaine baron in the Americas during the mid-1990s — apparently carked it while undergoing liposuction and cosmetic surgery at Mexico City's Santa Monica hospital, the country's response was to look for a set-up. The patient had checked in under the name of Antonio Flores Montes and the bruised and surgically scarred corpse was simply assumed to be some convenient victim hauled in as Carrillo's dead body double. This was not the view of the chief surgeon, who promptly fled the country. Neither was it the opinion of the DEA, FBI or the Mexican police — all of whom declared fingerprint and DNA analysis as conclusive proof that the cadaver was Carrillo. Champagne corks must have popped in Washington DC that night.

The trouble is that killing cartel leaders — even big fish like Carrillo — makes not a jot of difference to cocaine street sales. The DEA admits as much in its website analysis of leading Colombian and Mexican traffickers. 'Until recently, the Colombian trafficking organizations, collectively known as the Cali mafia, dominated the international cocaine market. Although some elements of the Cali mafia continue to play an important role in the world's wholesale cocaine market, events in recent years — including the

> **Mexico increased its cocaine seizures from 7.6 tonnes/tons in the first four months of 2000 to 10.7 tonnes/tons in the same period for 2001 — a 40 per cent increase.** White House Office of National Drug Control Policy, 5 October 2001

capture of the Rodriguez-Orejuela brothers in 1995, the death of Jose Santacruz-Londono in March 1996 and the surrender of Pacho Herrera in September 1996 — have accelerated the decline of the Cali mafia influence.

'Other experienced traffickers, who have been active for years but worked in the shadow of the Cali drug lords, have successfully seized opportunities to increase their share of the drug trade ... Independent Colombian traffickers are still responsible for most of the world's cocaine production and wholesale distribution.'

This is the problem for western governments. For every cocaine godfather taken down, six more are clamouring to nab his markets. It's the same with the drug couriers. As police and customs technology gets better, so the smuggling gets sneakier.

DELIVERING THE GOODIES

Smuggling is the frontline of the 'war on drugs'. You've perhaps heard politicians talk about this war as if there's a clear enemy, maybe a Mexican with 'Search Me, I'm A Smuggler' emblazoned on his T-shirt. Not many Mexicans try that one. There are too many other ways to get rich running cocaine without gambling on a double-bluff.

Here's the scale of the problem facing the United States Customs Service (USCS). According to its own statistics, 60 million people arrive in America on more than 675,000 commercial and private flights each year. Another 370 million come by land and 6 million by sea. Around 116 million vehicles cross the land borders with Canada and Mexico. Upwards of 90,000 merchant and passenger ships enter American ports carrying a combined total of 9 million shipping containers and 400 million tonnes/tons of cargo. In addition, 157,000 smaller vessels visit the harbours of coastal towns. Would *you* know the enemy? Exactly.

A quick tally reveals 436 million people arriving every year. The vast majority are good, decent law-abiding citizens but the task of picking out the bad guys falls to just 7,500 USCS officers at 301 ports of entry. The odds are not great but the USCS, the US Coast Guard, the Navy, DEA, FBI and CIA undoubtedly do disrupt drug smuggling effectively. There are 26 customs jets on interdiction deployment with smuggler 'host countries'. Customs P3 aircraft mount continuous surveillance over the Andean mountains to identify potential drug planes, and over the eastern Pacific to spot suspicious inbound ships. Fast Coast Guard cutters patrol the Caribbean and Pacific trafficking corridors.

Of the 86,700kg (190,000lbs) of cocaine seized in the USA during the fiscal year 2001, 40,000kg (88,000lbs) was being taken across the US/Mexican border. It's easy to see why. The border is mostly desert, unpopulated, unpatrolled, unfenced, and stretches for 3,200km

(2,000 miles). The US government does its best with radar balloons and the odd surveillance aircraft but, frankly, you could march a couple of battalions across before anyone noticed. Most smugglers still use the tarmac roads but as there aren't very many of these, congestion causes a different set of problems. At the entry point of San Ysidro, south of San Diego, 20,000 pedestrians and 96,000 car passengers travel across the world's busiest land border post every day.

Among the hi-tech gadgets used by customs officers to monitor this mass of humanity is something called a 'density-buster' – a kind of ultrasound scanner that can tell, for instance, whether your tyres contain more than just air. Digital cameras photograph 40,000 car registration plates a day, simultaneously checking them against national databases of suspect cars. On the USA side, metal tyre shredders can be raised, *Thunderbirds*-style, from the road to stop drivers crashing through inspection booths. But the best way of rooting out cocaine stashes is to use the most unbelievably sensitive drug-odour detectors known to man: dogs.

In March 2001 one attempt to keep sniffer mutts at bay involved packing 1,000kg (2,200lbs) of cocaine into a trailer carrying pallets of onions. It was stopped by police in rural Hidalgo County on the Texas/Mexico border and escorted to the Pharr port of entry for examination. The powerful smell of the onions didn't seem to worry sniffer dog Scar who immediately alerted them to the presence of drugs.

Customs officers tell stories of wised-up traffickers vacuum-sealing cocaine, smearing the package in grease, sealing it again and sinking it into a car petrol tank. Doesn't work. Dogs such as German shepherds – one of several breeds used by the USCS – have 220 million sensory cells in their noses, compared to just five million in humans. They can thoroughly check a car in six minutes. Even a cursory search by officers would take 20.

GO CREATE!
Tried and trusted smuggling methods include false compartments in suitcases and aerosol spray cans, false soles in shoes, swallowing 'bullets' (small amounts of coke wrapped in plastic or condoms and swallowed),

solutions of cocaine in wine or brandy bottles, baby powder containers – the list goes on. But as detection techniques are improving, smugglers are having to think more creatively. On 26 February 2001, customs special agents raided a bungalow in Nogales, Arizona, where they found a 7.5m (25ft) long hand-dug tunnel linked to the city's sewer system. Given that 198 cocaine bricks were found in the front room, and that Mexico lay three-quarters of a mile to the south, it's clear what was happening.

THE HIGH SEAS

American successes on land are more than matched by results at sea. In 2000 and 2001 there was a string of record-breaking marine seizures involving cocaine. Using boats is a huge gamble for traffickers because it's obviously impossible to spread risk. You can send 100 drug mules through an airport and if two-thirds make it the losses are manageable. But if your boat gets busted, it's painful – even for a cartel boss.

Yet moving cocaine by sea seems as popular as ever, at least if seizure figures announced by the White House Office of National Drug Control Policy are any guide. In October 2001 its acting director Edward Jurith revealed that 62,800kg (138,334lbs) of the drug was recovered by US Coast Guard vessels over the previous 12 months – almost 2,700kg (6,000lbs) more than the previous record (set the previous year). This can mean one of three things:

1 the Coast Guard is getting better or luckier;
2 there's more cocaine on the ocean;
3 both of the above.

Jurith had no doubt that pooling international resources was the key. He told a Washington DC press conference (5 October 2001) that, 'This increase in seizures takes place at the same time that other data tell us US consumers are using an ever-smaller proportion of the world's cocaine. Seizing more from a smaller universe of drugs is exactly what supply reduction aims to do. Much of the success is due to international cooperation, information-sharing and targeted operations. Foreign governments are also doing better – and for many of the same reasons.'

Of the 2001 successes, by far the greatest was the boarding of the Belize-flagged fishing boat *Svesda Maru* on 3 May 2001. This 45m (150ft) vessel was first sighted on 28 April by one of US Customs' P3 aircraft. Its position in the eastern Pacific was reported the following day by a Coast Guard C-130 patrol plane, and a decision was made to despatch a US Navy Guided Missile Frigate carrying specialist search teams. After five days they discovered a large, unexplained area beneath the fish holds – at least it was unexplained until they found a 12,000kg (26,400lbs) stash of cocaine. This single seizure was the biggest in maritime history, equivalent to one-sixteenth of the entire cocaine haul confiscated on mainland America that year.

> A Haitian man aroused suspicion when he arrived at Miami International Airport wearing a bulky plaster cast on his supposedly broken arm. Under questioning he changed his story several times and was taken to hospital to have the cast removed. Around 1kg (2¼lbs) of cocaine was discovered inside. *New York Times*, 28 February 2001

It wasn't just American agencies that broke seizure records in 2001. On 27 July Federal Police recovered Australia's largest single cocaine consignment soon after it was offloaded from a 30m (100ft) fishing boat in Dulverton Bay, a remote stretch of the western Australian coast some 650km (400 miles) north of Perth. Around 1,000kg (2,200lbs) of cocaine were buried on a lonely beach and soon afterwards the boat sank in what police euphemistically called 'inexplicable circumstances'. Five people were arrested.

In March 2002 it was the British government's turn to celebrate. After a joint surveillance operation and raid by Her Majesty's Customs & Excise and the National Crime Squad (NCS), five marine traffickers were jailed for a total of 99 years. They had been caught red-handed offloading 400kg (880lbs) of cocaine to a safe house on the Isle of Wight, off southern England. This, too, was a record cocaine seizure.

It was also a good illustration of the way anti-trafficking agencies turn vague rumours into hard intelligence. British Customs officers had their suspicions about gang leader Michael Tyrrell, an apparently wealthy individual with no obvious means of support. In July 2000 they received a tip-off that he was planning 'something big' and co-launched Operation Eyeful with the NCS, placing 55-year-old Tyrrell under round-the-clock surveillance. They knew he'd bought a £650,000 ($950,000) property complete with private beach on the Isle of Wight and in September they discovered he had acquired an 11m (37ft) yacht called the *Blue Hen*, which was moored in the Caribbean.

The yacht, crewed by two Frenchmen (Laurent Penchef and Didier Le Brun) and a Colombian (Herman Henao), was tracked across the Atlantic until it arrived off the Isle of Wight on 22 October. By now, a welcoming party of 150 Customs men was securely hidden in undergrowth, but initially the trap couldn't be sprung. Penchef and Henao had set off for shore in an inflatable dinghy, only to suffer engine failure. This coincided with an unforgiving English Channel storm, and the hapless pair were forced to take up oars, landing their coke a mile away from the agreed rendezvous point on Tyrrell's private beach.

They were met by their furious boss and his American sidekick, Robert Kavanagh. The five men then spent hours carrying the £90 million ($130 million) haul along a treacherous clifftop path back to Tyrrell's house, only to find themselves surrounded as they brought in the final bales. Sentencing the men at Snaresbrook Cown Court, London, in March 2002, Judge Timothy King told them, 'Drug smuggling is a scourge on our society. The clear message I send out today to other traffickers of drugs and addictive substances is one of zero tolerance.'

LET'S WORK TOGETHER …

As Ed Jurith pointed out, anti-drug agencies across the globe have increasingly been pooling resources and sharing intelligence. This would have been unthinkable a few decades ago, given the underlying suspicion that existed even between political allies. But the trafficking business recognizes no borders and so 'inter-agency partnership' is now the buzz-phrase from Miami to Frankfurt. The end of the Cold War has also been a factor. With the USA and Europe now pally with the Russians, foreign intelligence agencies can point their radio mikes and spy cameras at drug smugglers.

So it was when, in June 1997, two international traffickers – Briton Tony Lavene and Bolivian Rene Black – met a successful British businesswoman called Patricia McMahon in a hotel near Lima, Peru, news soon filtered back to Customs HQ in London. As the senior investigation officer, Martin Wilson, later told the London *Daily Telegraph* (2 April 1999), 'Two known drug runners and McMahon – it was something we decided to have a look at and from that point we were alerted to their activities.'

And what activities. Tricia McMahon, then aged 49, ran a successful public relations company whose client list included the British round-the-world yachtswoman Tracey Edwards MBE. Her husband was former European showjumping champion Paddy McMahon and the two of them mixed easily among the wealthy South American polo set. In this way Tricia was introduced to Black and, through him, to Lavene. Lavene had just completed a 14-year sentence for running cocaine. Tricia was going through a marriage hiatus and fell for him. They began a passionate affair.

Customs officers staking out her exclusive one-bedroom flat in Chelsea, London, could hardly miss the action.

> Police in Lausanne, Switzerland, arrested 1,175 African cocaine dealers in 2001 – more than double the previous year's tally. The ancient city has become a magnet for asylum-seekers who trade cocaine professionally. Possession of 0.2g or less is not an offence under Swiss law. *Time Europe* magazine, 18 March 2002

Video cameras and listening devices recorded the lovers snorting cocaine and indulging in marathon orgies. It must have been a belting assignment for the watchers although, sadly, the footage is unlikely ever to reach your local Odeon.

'It was the height of hedonism; drug-taking and four-in-a-bed sex, sometimes homosexual and sometimes heterosexual,' a Customs source told the *Daily Telegraph*. 'It was the classic sex, drugs and rock'n'roll. And I don't suppose their partners ever knew what was going on.'

Unlike HM Customs. They knew that Tricia McMahon paid for her flat in cash – £350 ($500) a week. They knew her landlord had been ordered not to forward mail to her marital home in Oxfordshire. They knew that her husband's horse-dealing business was in trouble. They knew she would want to maintain her glitzy lifestyle. And so they eavesdropped on Tricia, Lavene and various accomplices at fashionable wine bars, west London cafés and quiet country pubs. The plan wasn't difficult to unravel. It involved smuggling 17kg (37lbs) of cocaine from Peru to Heathrow Airport hidden in two tons of best-quality Peruvian asparagus. And to carry on doing this throughout the Peruvian asparagus season.

The first cocaine consignment arrived on 19 July 1998. It was handled by a crooked freight warehouseman and driven to a caravan park at nearby Henley-on-Thames. Several of the gang were arrested there. Lavene was pulled at his caravan in Poole, Dorset. And when Tricia McMahon returned from a short break in Venice with her blissfully unaware husband, Customs officers were waiting at passport control. She got 12 years. At the time of writing Lavene is a fugitive from justice. While awaiting trial he walked out of Wandsworth Prison, south London, wearing a prison warder's uniform and hasn't been seen since.

McMahon hardly fits the stereotypical image of an international drugs trafficker. She didn't surround herself with muscle and she never got caught up in gunfights. She was a PR person, an image creator, a lady who lunches. But if you think she was an unlikely suspect then what about Laurie Hiett, wife of American army colonel James Hiett. His job was to command anti-cocaine operations in Colombia during the late 1990s. Hers, it seems, was to ship some back home.

Laurie was jailed for five years in May 2000 after she admitted sending $700,000-worth (£480,000) of the drug from Bogotá to New York via the American Embassy diplomatic bag. Her husband denied direct involvement but later pleaded guilty to a federal charge of knowing that she'd laundered drug money. He also applied for retirement.

In an interview with the CBS *60 Minutes* programme (5 May 2000) Laurie said, 'I had this pound ... of pure cocaine underneath my jacuzzi and it was never ending. I was just doing it and doing it ... It was making me crazy ... It was so beautiful.' She blamed the army for sending her to Colombia even though senior officers knew she had a history of cocaine abuse. She had received rehabilitation treatment at a military hospital, but when challenged about this her husband assured his superiors that 'She's fine, she can do it, she hasn't done drugs since '95.'

The likes of Laurie Hiett and Tricia McMahon are never going to be major conduits for cocaine distribution. They were essentially opportunists; women thrust into the drugs trade through fate and circumstance. People like them come and go. But the really big trafficking organizations need regular, reliable courier systems in which loss risk is spread and transport is always secure. This is why air passengers – the ubiquitous drug mules touched upon in the previous chapter – are in such demand. Wholesalers know roughly what percentage will get through. They just factor it into their profit margins.

But what happens when the percentages change? When suddenly everyone is getting searched and flights are delayed or cancelled? When American port-of-entry officers work 16-hour days to make sure no smuggler gets an easy ride. Under these circumstances – post-11 September 2001 circumstances – tactics have to be reviewed. And among air traffickers, at least, they changed.

CRACKDOWN

Three months after the attacks on the World Trade Center and the Pentagon, US Customs Commissioner Robert Bonner pointed out that America's war on terrorism was also bad news for traffickers. 'Contrary to what some might believe, the counter-terrorism and counter-narcotics missions are not mutually exclusive,' he said. 'One does not necessarily come at the expense of the other. Everyone … knows that there is a nexus between drug trafficking and terrorism. Everyone in Colombia knows this' (speech to the 2001 National High Intensity Drug Trafficking Areas (HIDTA) conference, Washington DC, 6 December 2001).

The tightening of America's domestic security briefly took its toll on land-based Mexican and Colombian cocaine operations. Cross-border runs were delayed as the underworld waited for things to calm down. 'In the end they got fed up waiting and carried on regardless,' USCS officer Dean Boyd told me. 'We saw cocaine seizures pick up in the fall of 2001 and early 2002. This was partly because we were deploying more people to counter terrorism along our borders. [The events of] 11 September did disrupt road trafficking – but not for long. We soon saw cocaine smugglers back down their usual routes. They knew, and we knew, that they had buyers waiting.'

For the air mules it was a different story. Before 11 September, 50 per cent of all drugs found on passengers arriving in the USA came from flights originating in Jamaica. Given that the island generates less than 3 per cent of US air traffic, this is some achievement. However, after the terrorist attacks, getting drugs through American airports became a nightmare. There was a sense that US air authorities had been too complacent in the past and they sure as hell weren't about to make the same mistake again. In Jamaica supplies built up. European markets, with their traditional high prices and expanding street dealerships, suddenly seemed more attractive than ever.

Superintendent Gladstone Wright of the Jamaican Constabulary Narcotics Division put it like this: 'In terms of what is happening in Britain, the trade has escalated sharply since 11 September. The couriers who would normally be travelling to America are unable to get their drugs through because security at the borders has become so tight. Cocaine is stockpiling in Jamaica and that is no good for the dealers. There is no viable market for the drug here. So it is all being diverted to Britain.

Crack cocaine sold for between $3 (£7) and $50 (£35) per rock in the US during 2000. The general range was between $10 (£7) and $20 (£14). Rocks varied in weight from a tenth to half a gram. *Drug Trafficking In The United States*, Drug Enforcement Administration, September 2001

'Becoming a drug mule is the most readily available form of employment in this country at the moment. It is a job that you do not need to be interviewed for, or have any kind of qualifications, but you can earn more money than most Jamaicans see in a lifetime. The economy here is very bad at the moment and unemployment among women is running at 22 per cent. These people are easy prey for the dealers' (London *Observer*, 6 January 2002).

The Netherlands' Schiphol Airport has become another key destination for British and European distribution. Police estimate that between 20,000 and 25,000 mules pass through the terminal each year, most of them Dutch citizens flying on return tickets from the former Caribbean colonies of the Antilles and Surinam. Government figures for 2001 show that 1,200 air passengers were convicted of cocaine trafficking, a 60 per cent increase on the previous year. Those who escaped arrest and made their delivery would have been paid around £2,000 ($2,900) plus expenses.

The situation at Schiphol got so bad after 11 September that, in January 2002, senior customs officers wrote a letter to the Amsterdam daily newspaper *Het Parool* complaining that they'd been ordered to stop arresting cocaine traffickers. The reason? Dutch jails were too full to take any more felons. This was despite the fact that during random checks on one flight from the Caribbean, no fewer than 40 smugglers had been caught. 'At a time when our society is being flooded with drugs,' the customs team wrote, 'we are being forced on the express orders of our superiors to stick our heads in the sand.'

They recounted one ludicrous case in which a woman found with 14kg (30lb) of coke in her luggage was released because no cell was available for her. Her £460,000 ($666,000) consignment was confiscated but she demanded – and got – a police receipt to prove to her drugs masters that she hadn't sold off the goodies herself.

HARD TO SWALLOW?

Of all the mules, the 'body packers' adopt the most ignominious technique. They prepare for their ordeal by swallowing whole grapes. Shortly before their flight they switch to compressed cocaine encased in the severed finger pieces of latex rubber gloves. These are sealed into pellets by a special machine and coated with honey to help prevent gagging. The sealing part of the process isn't quite perfect. This is probably why at least ten mules died of cocaine poisoning during 2001 while waiting to board flights at Kingston Airport.

Once the pellets are swallowed (payment is per pellet and swallowers are believed to manage anywhere between 30 and 120 in a single sitting) the mule will take a large dose of anti-diarrhoea tablets to induce constipation. After the flight there's then a six-day wait for nature to take its course. It's a shitty way to make a living but, hey, at least it's *their* shit.

Let me guess what you're thinking. How did it come to this? How did supposedly civilized societies reduce their citizens to swallowing rubber gloves filled with chemically laden drugs to be crapped out and handed to others to mix with yet more chemicals so that different people would pay big bucks to snort or smoke them and feel cool? I mean, you couldn't make it up. All this nonsense over one ordinary little plant.

Time for a history lesson.

HISTORY

> 'I have been reading about cocaine, the essential constituent of coca leaves, which some Indian tribes chew to enable them to resist privations and hardships. A German has been employing it with soldiers and has in fact reported that it increases their energy and capacity to endure. I am procuring some myself.'
>
> – Sigmund Freud, in a letter, 21 April 1884

FOOD OF THE GODS

Who knows how it happened – how the very first South American became the very first coke-head. It would have been several thousand, maybe tens of thousands of years ago, that this 'First User' would have ripped off a bunch of coca leaves and taken a tentative chew to check out the taste.

Suppose this Indian – let's call him/her Charlie for obvious and convenient reasons – tried to improve the flavour and texture by adding a touch of alkali. This could have been burned roots, powdered lime, sea shells or anything else in the native diet with a high pH. Alkalis like these leach out the rush-giving alkaloids from coca.

There's no doubt that over the next few hours this primitive equivalent of chewing gum would have made Charlie feel cool about, say, hunting guanaco for that day's dinner. It wouldn't have matched the coked-up buzz enjoyed by today's users as most coca leaves contain less than 1 per cent cocaine. To get a 21st-century-style high Charlie would have had to dry the leaves, pound them up and consume 50g-worth (1¾oz) in one mega-snort.

Even so, the leaves would have produced a gradual onset of euphoria and well-being, a marked lack of hunger and fatigue, and heightened mental alertness.

If advertising and entrepreneurial instincts had existed in those days, Charlie would surely have marketed his product as The Hunter's Friend. But they didn't, so he just told everyone the great news. Within a few generations coca would have progressed in Indian culture from unremarkable shrub to food of the gods.

This version of events is admittedly light on fact. But, in essence, it is true. South American Indians were the first people to use coca simply because it didn't grow anywhere else. It has become a defining part of their culture, helps them work longer and harder, performs wonders as an anaesthetic (the Inca seemed very keen on it for brain surgery), treats snow blindness, stomach upsets, headaches and altitude sickness, and even, so it turns out, provides some useful nutrition.

COCA ROOTS

Coca is a member of the genus *Erythroxylum*, of which there are around 250 species, mostly native to South America and all heavily reliant on wet, frost-free, warm, humid growing conditions. It grows faster at sea level but its cocaine yield increases at altitude and most commercial plantations are found at heights between 450 and 1,800m (1,500 and 6,000ft). As a result, the continent's prime cocaine belt runs from Colombia in the north, down the eastern foothills of the Andes to southern Bolivia and the eastern edge of the Amazon basin. Many, though not all, species contain cocaine although only a few contain enough to make cultivation worth the candle. Of these few, four in particular have cornered the market.

- *Erythroxylum coca* **variety** *coca*. Usually known as Bolivian coca, this was for many years the biggest source of illegal cocaine. It still plays a major role in Bolivia's agricultural economy and, according to the United Nations Drug Control Programme, the country's total annual harvest is currently around 93,000 tonnes/tons.
- *Erythroxylum novogranatense* **variety** *novogranatense*. This one is native to Colombia – a region known as Nueva Granada (New Granada) to Spanish colonists – hence the plant's name. This was the first coca leaf seen by white Europeans and its cocaine was later exported all over the world as a legal, medical anaesthetic. For years it never much

featured in international trafficking; at least not until the big Colombian cartels decided during the 1980s that they could expand profit margins by growing their own instead of importing from Bolivia and Peru. It was a canny move, given that *novogranatense* now services 85 per cent of the world's illegal cocaine market.

■ *Erythroxylum novogranatense* variety *truxillense*. Better known as Trujillo this flourishes in the dry, coastal desert strip around the Peruvian city of the same name. Because of the climate, Trujillo can only grow in well-irrigated plantations but its flavoursome leaves and high cocaine content made it well worth the effort for Inca tribes who knew it as 'Royal Coca'. Mother Nature gets particularly motherly where Trujillo is concerned because its cocaine content is a total nightmare to extract commercially. For this reason it has never been much use to traffickers, although it is the leaf of choice for the manufacturers of Coca-Cola. In case you were wondering, coca leaves are still used to give Coca-Cola its flavour – but only *after* the cocaine has been removed. So when right-wing politicians and middle-aged golfers finger-wag you at drinks parties and demand to know why the world coca crop can't just be blitzed by the CIA you can tell them the truth. It's to keep the world's greatest soft drink up there as market leader. Besides, Bacardi doesn't taste as good on its own.

■ *Erythroxylum coca* variety *ipadu*. Another coca variety which, until the last two decades, rarely interested traffickers because of its fairly low cocaine count. It is native to the Amazon basin and has been chewed by Indians there for aeons. The war on drugs and drug plantations by western governments has increasingly forced growers to look to *ipadu* and the Amazon as a safer, discreet source.

A DIRECT LINE TO THE PAST

There are two sources for the history of coca – archaeological (still somewhat patchy) – and written, which begins when Francisco Pizarro and his conquistador cronies tipped up to conquer the Inca in 1532. For many years the prehistoric archaeology of South America was dominated by a view that human occupation began well after 18,000 BC, when an Ice Age

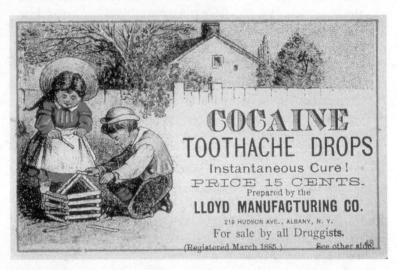

Advertisement from around 1885 for cocaine toothache drops, featuring two children playing happily. The drug was first isolated from the leaves of the coca plant in 1855 and thereafter became widely used as a local anaesthetic, but its use was subsequently restricted due to its addictive nature.

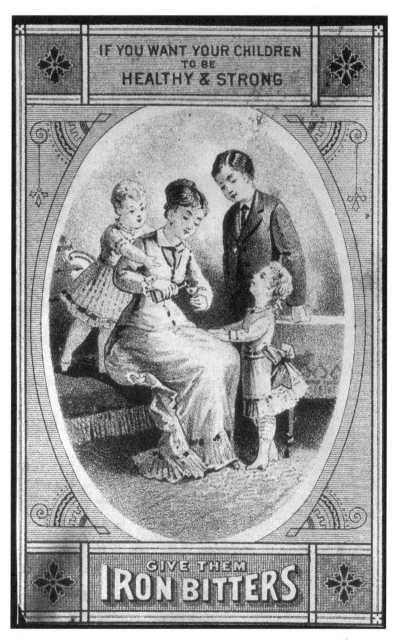

Brown's Iron Bitters, a patented medicine containing cocaine, was claimed to cure malaria, dyspepsia, and 'female infirmities', and was even promoted (as shown here) as a general tonic for children. Popular in the USA, Iron Bitters was prevalent until strict legislation was introduced in the early 20th century.

Arctic land bridge allowed Asian migrants to colonize what are now Alaska and Canada. The theory was supported by the carbon dating of tools and weapons of the Stone Age Clovis people, whose cultures were widespread further south, to around 10,000 BC.

Then, in 1977, discoveries at Monte Verde, Southern Chile, by the American archaeologist Tom Dillehay turned all this on its head. Radiocarbon tests showed that much of the material he unearthed was laid down in 11,000 BC, opening the possibility that hunter-gatherer people were living in the southern Andes as early as 31,000 BC.

The Monte Verde tribe's religion was apparently important enough for labour to be assigned to the construction of a ritual temple. It had

> The pharmaceutical company Merck, of Darmstadt, Germany, produced a total of 50g (1¾oz) of cocaine for commercial use in 1879. Some of this was used by Sigmund Freud in his early experiments. By 1906 Merck's output had risen to 4 tonnes/tons per year.

gravel footings, wooden stakes strengthening its walls and a central platform. Here Dillehay's team found remnants of medicinal plants (though not coca) – an indication that the temple was used for healing ceremonies as well as perhaps ancestor worship.

The word coca is thought by many anthropologists to derive from *khoka*, which literally meant 'the plant' in the tongue of the pre-Incan Tiwanaku people. Centred on Lake Titicaca, this culture developed a highly efficient agricultural system in which raised beds and shoreline canals lengthened the growing season. For these farmers to christen coca *the* plant – as opposed to any old plant – gives some idea of their regard for it. Tiwanaku dates from at least the third century AD, declining around AD 1000, and its legacy is the Quechuan language spoken by ten million people from Ecuador to Argentina.

By the time the Inca arrived on the scene, coca production had really taken off. The Inca were a remarkable people. They transformed themselves from a 12th-century minor tribe confined to a 30km (20 mile) radius of Cuzco, in Peru's Cordillera region, to become masters of an empire stretching for some 3,500km (2,175 miles) north to south and 800km (500 miles) east to west. And they achieved all this in under 100 years.

It was the eighth Inca (ie emperor) Viracocha who began seizing new territory in 1437. But it was his son Pachacuti, grandson Topa and great-grandson Huayna Capac who really caught the empire-building bug. By the time Huayna died in 1525 Inca influence stretched from what is now southern Colombia, through Ecuador and Peru and on to Bolivia, northern Argentina and Chile – a total population of anything up to 16 million.

Their power was rooted in natural aggression and superb organization. The fact that people worshipped the emperor as a living god certainly helped – no wishy-washy democracy here. Good communications across the empire were crucial - the four administrative areas were linked by a 24,000km (15,000 mile) network of stone roads, tunnels and vine suspension bridges. These were reserved for teams of state-appointed messengers capable of covering 400km (250 miles) per day. Food production was organized on rigid communist lines, with government experts choosing crops, supervising irrigation, terracing and fertilization, and taking a share of the harvest to store in times of need. A healthy percentage of this would have been coca. In fact, coca was key to the whole shebang. It was the centre of religious life.

Inca religion regarded the leaf as divine and magical. Priests used it for offerings, chewed it during rituals (and in the presence of the emperor), burnt it to ensure its glorious aroma pleased the gods, scattered its ashes to keep the fertility goddess Pachamama happy and placed it with the dead to stop spirits returning to the land of the living.

Predicting the future was part of a high priest's job and if there was one thing Inca folk liked in a priest it was divination. Oracles were tapped up over everything from sickness to criminal investigations and, most importantly, the timing of sacrifices. Conclusions could be drawn from simple rituals – watching the path of a spider in an upturned bowl – to messier ones such as inspecting the marks on sacrificed llama lungs. Inevitably, coca was right up there as a divination aid. Leaves would be flung into the air or thrown on to liquid and 'read' according to how they landed.

Daily offerings to Inca deities were common, but animal or human sacrifices were saved for special occasions or to limit the threat of flood, disease or famine. It is thought that hundreds of children were killed to mark the accession of an Inca emperor, and individuals were occasionally singled out as special emissaries to the gods. We know this because one boy, sacrificed on Mount Aconcagua late in the 15th century, has been found preserved in the 5,300m (17,550ft) permafrost.

The corpse bore no sign of violence and there was no obvious cause of death. His face was smeared with a red pigment, he wore two embroidered tunics, a turquoise necklace, plumed head-dress, and sandals. He carried gold and shell ornaments shaped as humans and animals, and thorny oyster shells from the Ecuador coast. Inevitably, coca leaves were carried in bags attached to the figures. Forensic analysis has shown that the child was not permitted to use them as he awaited his fate.

Just as it featured in death ritual, so coca was celebrated as symbolic of life. Young men from high-ranking families would sometimes undergo a fearsome initiation into manhood, which could involve flogging, racing and sparring. More commonly this rite of passage took the form of a simple race in which the final straight was lined by young women making suggestive quips and offering coca or *chicha* (weak beer). Finishers, or survivors, were rewarded with a sling and a coca pouch marking their emergence into manhood. Even today, one Colombian tribe still practises an initiation ritual in which candidates 'marry' the coca leaf.

Perhaps because of its special place in Inca society, some historians have argued that coca was restricted to an elite. There's no doubt that it was, literally, close to the heart of the Inca (emperor) himself, because the only object he ever carried was the coca pouch around his neck. Two emperors even named their wives after the leaf, using the sacred title *Mama Coca*. Only two other crops were credited with the *Mama* prefix – maize and cinchona.

Other important state officials would have been allocated coca rations as a perk or necessity of the job – priests, doctors, magicians, warriors, leaders of defeated tribes, memorizers of state records (the Inca never bothered with writing) and those fleet-footed messengers. This is not to say that ordinary people were banned from using it. Given that coca had been around for millennia before the Inca, this would have been a hopeless task. Besides, why ban it? Judging by the huge plantations in the Huánuco Valley and at Yungas in Bolivia there was no shortage. Far more sensible to concentrate on controlling production and distribution, much in the style of the Chilean government before General Pinochet.

Traditional methods of consuming coca have continued unchanged since Charlie and co (see above) first got high. A user grabs a few leaves from his personal coca pouch or *chuspa*, wedges them between his teeth and cheek and starts working in a bit of saliva. Then he takes out his *iscupuru*, a gourd containing a concentrated, highly caustic alkaline like powdered shells or roots, and removes a smidgen with a stick.

This powder, known as *llipta* to the Indians, is then carefully pushed into the middle of the coca wad, raising pH levels in the mouth and increasing the speed with which cocaine alkaloids are leached out of the leaf wad. There's a bit of a knack to it. You're not so much chewing as occasionally manipulating the wad with your tongue to keep it moist and exposed to saliva. And one slip with your *llipta* and you've got an internal mouth burn that makes the world's hottest madras feel like cold yoghurt. To guard against this, Indian mothers introducing their children to coca will often 'mix' the *llipta* themselves before transferring it to the child's mouth.

The most obvious effect is that your saliva turns bright green. However, you tend not to worry about this because your mouth is already tingling pleasantly and your throat feels like it's having an out-of-body experience. You have no interest in food and you feel ready to hit the road running. It is by all accounts a far less intense rush then you'd get snorting a line in your neighbourhood club toilets but because the coca is releasing alkaloids gradually, this 'slow rush' persists for much longer.

There is, incidentally, a continuing medical debate about whether the South American chewer, or *coqueros*, are unreconstructed coke addicts or simply 'social' chewers – much in the way western medics will argue the toss about social drinking and alcoholism. Some say your typical *coqueros* has a daily intake of around 15mg, that's about the amount of caffeine in a strong cup of coffee. Others reckon it's closer to half a gram of pure cocaine, which in western street terms is a hefty habit. There is all sorts of sophistry in this kind of debate, but one thing is certain. To a *coqueros*, coca is as much a part of life as a cold beer is to a steel worker. Two different cultures. Two different drugs. Same outrage if anyone suggests a ban.

COCA AND THE CONQUISTADORS

One of the great things about the Spanish (and if you were an Inca Indian there weren't many) is that their explorers in the Americas kept detailed diaries. These reveal fascinating early impressions of coca, including the one reprinted below, which was noted down during the fourth voyage of Christopher Columbus, who sailed from Cadiz in May 1502. For various reasons that don't really concern us here, Columbus had been having a hard time, what with leaky, worm-ridden ships and an abortive attempt to find a westward sea passage through the new continent. He probably gave little thought to the account of one of his lieutenants returning from a river trip inland near Belem, the chief port of the lower Amazon. But he noted it all the same.

'The lieutenant went into the country with 40 men, a boat following with 40 more. The next day they came to the river Urisa, seven leagues west from Belem. The cacique [tribe leader] came a league out of the town to meet him with some 20 men and presented him with such things as they feed on and some gold plates were exchanged here. This cacique and his chief man never ceased putting dry herb into their mouths, which they chewed, and sometimes they took a sort of powder, which they carried along with that herb, which singular custom astonished our people very much.'

The Italian navigator Amerigo Vespucci was also baffled by coca. Vespucci is considered a bit of a fantasist by today's scholars (who doubt that he ever actually landed in North America as he claimed) but he did explore a large part of South America's northern coast and his name would later be used to christen both the new continents. He came across coca when he landed on the island of Santa Margarita, off Venezuela, in 1499 and was immediately revolted by the way its 'loathsome' people chewed it. In one letter, published five years later, he included the following report.

'They all had their cheeks swollen out with a green herb inside, which they were constantly chewing like beasts so they could scarcely utter speech: and each one had upon his neck two dried gourds, one of which was full of that herb, which they kept in their mouths and the other full of a white flour, which looked like powdered chalk and from time to time with a small stick, which they kept moistening in their mouths they dipped it into the flour and then put it into their mouths in both cheeks ... This they did very frequently. And, marvelling at such a thing, we were unable to comprehend their secret.'

Others were more positive. In 1609 Garcilaso de la Vega's classic account of the history and conquest of the Inca, *Royal Commentaries of Peru*, carried a priest's account of coca medicine. 'Our doctors use it in powdered form to reduce the swelling of wounds, to strengthen broken bones, to expel cold from the body or prevent it entering, and to cure rotten wounds or sores that are full of maggots. And if it does so much for outward ailments, will not its singular virtue have even greater effect in the entrails of those who eat it?'

THE COCA CONQUERORS

Vespucci was by no means the only European interested in this strange new world. Spanish adventurers were on the hunt for a fast buck – namely gold and silver – and they had the comfort of knowing that God was on their side. They knew this because the Pope had given them the Inca empire back in 1493, in a way that only Popes can. They therefore wasted no time in claiming vast territories for Spain and sending home horror stories of the un-Christian cannibals and barbarians who passed for human beings. This in turn provided a sensible reason to kill as many as possible, a task the Spanish embraced with enthusiasm. Yet they were outnumbered by hundreds of thousands of Inca warriors. How did it happen? How *could* it happen?

In fact, the Inca empire was on borrowed time from the moment it first encountered white Europeans.

> In 1548 a few thousand Bolivian silver miners were together chewing 100,000 *cestas* (baskets) of coca per year – more than 1 million kg (2.2 million lb). They relied on it to fend off thirst and hunger and to provide energy for working long shifts. At the time, 'addiction' would have been a meaningless concept.

The Indians had no natural immunity to the diseases imported by sailors – plague, smallpox and measles all probably figured – and, by 1527, something like 200,000 Inca had died. Among them was their most successful emperor, Huayna Capac.

The downfall of the Inca is a book in itself but, essentially, here's what happened. After Huayna Capac's death, one of his sons, Huascar, fought a civil war of accession against a half-brother, Atahualpa. Atahualpa emerged victorious but then discovered a new threat in the form of the Spanish conquistador Francisco Pizarro and his motley private army of 183 fortune-seekers.

Pizarro had got permission from Spain's Charles I to invade Peru in return for one-fifth of the booty. He landed on 15 November 1532 and arranged a parley with Atahualpa, who wasn't really expecting trouble but brought along 5,000 warriors just in case. Atahualpa was greeted at the rendezvous point by a priest who handed him a bible, asked if he believed in Christ and whether he accepted Charles I as his king. These were big questions and, predictably, Atahualpa passed on all three – hurling the bible to the ground. The priest then dived for cover shouting 'Fall on. I absolve you all.' At which point the hidden Spanish musketeers opened fire, killing 3,000 Inca in barely an hour while sustaining no serious casualties themselves.

Pizarro took Atahualpa prisoner and used him as a puppet ruler while he looted as much gold and silver as he could. Indoctrinated with the idea that the Inca's word was law, his people carried on their daily lives with little concern about the presence of occupying Spanish soldiers. Once Atahualpa's usefulness had expired he was summarily tried and garrotted, but for Pizarro the venture would ultimately end in disaster. With famine and disease raging across the land, he quarrelled with his fellow Spaniards and was assassinated in 1541.

In the big picture, Pizarro's death is meaningless. The Spanish were firmly in control – the only problem for them was to find something worth controlling. The rivers of gold they had expected to find were just not flowing and the only commodity the Indians really seemed to rate was this strange plant called coca.

CHEWING OVER THE POSSIBILITIES

Coca did nothing for the Spanish. Chewing was a revolting habit and you couldn't export the stuff – even if a European market existed – because it rotted so easily. That said, they were never ones to pass up a business opportunity and it seemed there was very little the Indians wouldn't do for coca. Gradually the settlers saw there was good money in plantations. Production went through the roof and the chewing habit spread even further than it had under the Inca.

Meanwhile, some Europeans began following up old legends about mountains that were made of silver. All these leads pointed to one place, Potosí, in what is now southern Bolivia, a mining area abandoned by the Inca after volcanic rumblings convinced them that the gods were angry. The Spanish had no such fears and when silver was rediscovered there in 1546 it was boom time. Inside a year a new city had been founded and 7,000 Indians were soon digging away, removing 70 tonnes/tons a year. Contemporary records suggest that in 1549 the Spanish crown's one-fifth share was something around 40,000 pesos per week. Potosí expanded exponentially until, by 1611, it had a population of 150,000. Yet all the time the mines got deeper and the Indians worked harder. They needed something that would sustain them. Guess what they chose ...?

In 1548 the miners of Potosí chewed their way through more than 1 million kg (almost 1,000 tons) of coca. Most wanted to be paid in coca (hard currencies such as the peso were a mystery to them) and so plantations pushed up production to meet demand. Everyone was getting rich, especially the mine owners. They sold silver ore to the smelters and overpriced coca to their workers. In 1553, the Spanish traveller Pedro Cieza de Leon described the trade as follows.

'Coca was taken to the mines of Potosí for sale, and the planting of the leaves and picking of the leaves was carried on to such an extent that coca is not now worth so much, but it will never cease to be valuable. There are some persons in Spain who are rich from the produce of this coca, having traded with it, sold and re-sold it in the Indian markets.'

The coca boom had its drawbacks and, predictably, it was the plantation workers that suffered the most. Even under the Inca the *cocalos* fields harboured parasitic diseases such as leishmaniasis, which can fatally damage internal organs and cause facial deformations. Under the Spanish boom, life expectancy in the fields was even lower.

Philip II of Spain was aware of this. He first ordered that no Indians be forced into the *cocalos*; then that they could work only for five months at a time. Both decrees were quietly ignored, but Philip knew that his ultimate sanction – banning coca production – would cause mayhem in the silver mines ... and therefore in his Treasury.

To fudge the issue he asked his new viceroy, Francisco de Toledo, to introduce some reforms. Toledo started well, enforcing labour restrictions on the plantation owners. But then he seized on the old Inca idea of a *mita* tax, under which all 1.6 million Indians between the ages of 18 and 50 would work every sixth year for the Spanish crown. On paper, *cocalos* conditions now looked good – proper salaries, two weeks off in every three, guaranteed land to grow food – but in practice they sucked. Salaries were cut, there were absurd production quotas and much of the workers' land was stolen by plantation bosses.

State slavery it may have been, but the *mita* produced results. It applied as much to silver miners as coca workers and over the next 200 years the Potosí complex would produce an astonishing 21,000 tonnes/tons. Throughout this time the Indians' lot grew steadily worse – shafts 300m (1,000ft) deep, miners scrambling around in unventilated tunnels with lighted candles bound to their thumbs and roof falls a daily hazard. It was the same in the newly discovered mercury mines at Huancavelica (mercury was crucial to a new, more efficient method of silver refining), except that there you could add cancer to the causes of death. In conditions like these, coca was the only way to get through the shift.

HOLIER THAN THOU?

While Spain counted her cash, the Roman Catholic Church got increasingly stuffy about the coca business. The First Council of Lima in 1552 heard talk of the plant as the Devil's work and a form of idolatry, and demanded it be banned. With a smooth bit of spin-doctoring, Philip II's father, Charles I of Spain, absolutely agreed and absolutely refused. The Second Council had another go 15 years later, this time hearing that coca encouraged 'demonic influences' and made women infertile. Again the Crown looked the other way. By the time of the Third Council, Philip II had got the hint and agreed that the Church should take a 10 per cent cut of all coca sales. Suddenly priests were commenting on how useful the leaf was to labourers. And for the next 200 years coca and South America carried on pretty much as usual.

THE BOFFINS TAKE A TRIP

For European scientists – particularly botanists – this was a frustrating time. They were like children locked out of a sweetshop, desperate to get into the new continent and start classifying all its amazing new species. Unfortunately the Spanish were not well disposed to the idea of rival powers playing with their train set and it wasn't until the French botanist Joseph de Jussieu arrived in South America in November 1734 that progress was made.

Jussieu was a member of the first scientific mission to the new continent, headed by a talented mathematician called Charles-Marie de la Condamine. The scientists were escorted everywhere by two Spanish naval officers (in case they turned out to be spies) and the expedition was dogged by ill-fortune and bad luck. But Condamine did make one sensational discovery in the form of resin from the cahout-chou tree, better known these days as rubber. It was not until 1771 that Jussieu finally made it home to Paris. By then he had lost his mind, mostly because every time he managed to assemble a decent specimen collection in Peru it either got lost or was burned. Nevertheless he did bring some samples home, one of which was coca. In 1786 it was classified by the biologist Jean Chevalier de Lamarck as *Erythroxylum coca*. Now scientists knew what coca was. They just didn't know how it worked.

Biochemistry was, at this time, little more than pseudo-science. Biologists were beginning to look at the natural chemicals in plants as potential medicines; the hard bit was to isolate them. In 1803 the German apothecary FWA Setürner successfully extracted morphine from opium. Strychnine, quinine, caffeine, nicotine and atropine were discovered over the next 30 years and science began grouping these and other nitrogen-based organic compounds as 'alkaloids'. The problem with coca, as we already know, is that it was a nightmare to export. There was never enough good-quality leaf on which to experiment.

In 1859 the breakthrough came. The celebrated German organic chemist Friedrich Wöhler arranged for a colleague working in Peru to bring back a 13.5kg (30lb) bale of coca. He then handed this to one of his best students, Albert Niemann, who analyzed it for his PhD. Niemann's dissertation was titled dryly 'On A New Organic Base In The Coca Leaves' and went into some elaborate detail.

The crux of it is that he washed the leaves in 85 per cent alcohol with a little sulphuric acid, distilled the alcohol to leave a sticky residue, separated this into a resin and shook that repeatedly with bicarbonate of soda. The end result was a palmful of small, rod-shaped crystals. As all the other alkaloids ended in 'ine' Niemann thought it right to follow suit. He named his compound coca-ine.

Niemann died the following year, aged just 26, not realising the magnitude of what he had done. Initially, neither did anyone else in the scientific community, but when word spread about an Italian doctor called Paolo Mantegazza, who enthusiastically published the results of coca experiments on himself, eyebrows were raised. Mantegazza's paper, entitled 'Coca Experiences', told how after a dose of 12g (⅓oz) he began leaping over his desk and felt himself 'capable of jumping on my neighbours' heads'. After 54g (1½oz), chewed over an entire day, he was really buzzing.

'I sneered at all the poor mortals condemned to live in the valley of tears while I, carried on the wings of two leaves of coca, went flying through the spaces of 77,438 worlds, each more splendid than the one before. An hour later I was sufficiently calm to write these words with a steady hand: God is unjust because he made man incapable of sustaining the effects of coca all life long. I would rather live a life of ten years with coca than one of 100,000 (and here I inserted a line of zeros) without it.'

There is evidence that Adolf Hitler was developing a cocaine habit. According to one of his physicians, Dr Erwin Giesing, Hitler was given the drug in a ten per cent solution to treat sore throats. Soon he was demanding it all the time and Giesing eventually refused to increase his daily dose.

Gradually, doctors began to suspect cocaine had its uses. Another self-experimenter was none other than Sir Robert Christison, 78-year-old president of the British Medical Association. He told the *British Medical*

Journal that during two 24km (15 mile) rambles, attempted with and without coca, he felt a huge energy boost when using the leaf.

'I was surprised to find that all sense of weariness had vanished and that I could proceed not only with ease but with elasticity,' he said. Later, Sir Robert told how, after leading some students to the top of a 1,000m (3,280ft) Scottish mountain, he had chewed a little coca for the return trip.

'I at once felt that all fatigue was gone and I went down the long descent with an ease which felt like that which I used to enjoy in the mountainous rambles in my youth,' he noted. '... The chewing of coca not only removes extreme fatigue, but prevents it. Hunger and thirst are suspended; but eventually appetite and digestion are unaffected. No injury is sustained at the time or subsequently in occasional trials.'

THE FIRST COCAINE USERS

While the boffins were somewhat slow off the mark, big business quickly recognized cocaine's potential. Among the first entrepreneurs to exploit the mass market was a Corsican apothecary called Angelo Mariani, who in 1863 hit on the idea of mixing the drug with wine.

The taste was pleasant enough but the real advantage was that alcohol worked as a solvent, extracting cocaine alkaloids from the leaf. Soon everyone in polite society had heard of Vin Mariani, an unsurprising fact since its maker was a real media tart. He shamelessly promoted his product by sending freebies to celebrities and publishing their grateful responses. As a result, newspaper readers would see endorsements such as those reproduced below.

> '*I took the precaution of bringing a small flask of Mariani Wine along with me and it was a great help. Its energetic action sustained me during the crossing.*' - Louis Blériot after flying across the English Channel in July 1909

> '*Since a single bottle of Mariani's extraordinary coca wine guarantees a lifetime of 100 years, I shall be obliged to live until the year 2700! Well, I have no objections.*' - Jules Verne

And on it went. Thomas Edison hinted that Vin Mariani was just the drink for a budding inventor, the Lumière brothers – fresh from inventing the cinema – swore by it and HG Wells indicated in a caricatured self-portrait how it transformed his mood. US President William McKinley's secretary wrote thanking Mariani for a case of wine and assured him the that President was already a fan. Mariani, reckoning he was on to a good thing, was now frantically marketing everything from coca sore-throat lozenges to coca tea.

COCA UNDER THE MICROSCOPE
While all this was going on, science at last got its act together. A promising young Austrian research student called Sigmund Freud read about cocaine experiments carried out on Bavarian soldiers by a Dr Theodore Aschenbrandt. Aschenbrandt's idea was to look at military applications for the drug and, clearly, an army on wizzo marching powder would be, as early enemies of the Inca discovered, *some* army.

At the time, Freud was hoping to make his fortune from some sensational medical discovery. Unfortunately, the discovery element of this plan was proving a tad tricky. He had fallen desperately in love with a Viennese girl, Martha Bernay, and they were engaged to be married. But he needed to show her parents a healthy bank balance.

In Ernest Jones' 1953 biography, *The Life And Work Of Sigmund Freud*, there is a letter from him to Martha dated 21 April 1884, in which he noted: 'I have been reading about cocaine, the essential constituent of coca leaves which some Indian tribes chew to enable them to resist privations and hardships. A German has been employing it with soldiers and has in fact reported that it increases their energy and capacity to endure. I am procuring some myself and will try it with cases of heart disease and also of nervous exhaustion.'

The letter continues, 'Perhaps others are working at it; perhaps nothing will come of it. But I shall certainly try it and you know that when one perseveres sooner or later one succeeds. We do not need more than one such lucky hit for us to be able to think of setting up house.'

For Freud, cocaine was not that lucky hit. He clearly thought it was a wonderful drug (judging by the free samples he sent out to colleagues and friends) and he found it a great way to alleviate bouts of depression (of which he had many). However, it seems he loved it a little too much. The paper he produced later, 'About Coca', could almost have been written by a coke-head, talking of 'the most gorgeous excitement' shown by animals injected with the drug and referring to 'offerings' rather than 'doses'. It was not exactly scientific language.

IT'S A KNOCKOUT ...
Freud would go on to invent psychoanalysis and be generally considered one of the 20th century's most innovative – or barmy – thinkers, depending on your point of view. But the future of cocaine was entwined with the fate of a younger colleague, the medical student Carl Koller, with whom Freud had been cooperating in cocaine experiments. Koller was obsessed with finding better anaesthetics, particularly for eye surgery. Knocking out patients with ether was hopeless (a) because those in frail condition might never recover and (b) because in coming round patients often vomited violently, tearing fragile sutures.

Koller had noticed that when pure cocaine touched his lips it made them feel numb. He'd mentioned this to Freud with little response but when another colleague casually remarked that the new drug 'numbed the tongue' realisation dawned. Koller dashed to a nearby laboratory and immediately conducted experiments: first on the eyes of a frog and then on his own eyes. He found that after applying a cocaine solution he could touch the cornea with a pinhead and feel nothing. On 15 September 1884 his discovery of the world's first local anaesthetic was placed before an astounded audience at the Heidelberg Ophthalmological Society's annual convention. One of medicine's most challenging problems had been solved by a mere 27-year-old intern.

Sigmund Freud was frustrated by Koller's triumph but he soon had more important things to worry about. That same year he was attempting to provide pain relief for his great friend Dr Ernst von Fleischl-Marxow, who had an excruciating nerve condition. Fleischl-Marxow had resorted to morphine to help him sleep and had become addicted. Freud offered him cocaine as an alternative. Inside 20 days, Freud reported later, all trace of the morphine craving had vanished while 'no cocaine habituation set in; on the contrary, an increasing antipathy to the drug was unmistakenly evident'.

Of course, Freud was wrong. The morphine habit had simply been replaced by a cocaine habit, and in April 1885, barely a year after Fleischl-Marxow first tried the new drug, he was in bits and pieces. Freud discovered he was injecting a full gram of cocaine solution every day and suffered from fits and fainting. Worse, the patient experienced a horrendous physical ordeal in which he believed insects were crawling around underneath his skin. He would sit staring at an arm or leg for long periods trying to pinch one out. Fleischl-Marxow was in fact suffering hallucinations caused by cocaine toxosis – the dreaded 'coke bugs'.

To his horror, Freud realised that he had produced the world's first cocaine addict. He began warning friends – particularly his beloved Martha – that they should now be extremely careful with the samples he'd sent them. What he did not know was that Fleischl-Marxow had also created a piece of social history by inventing the 'speedball', a dose of cocaine and morphine (or heroin) taken simultaneously.

He found that the stimulant effects of cocaine worked well alongside the 'downer' offered by morphine and that this combination taken intravenously helped get him through the day. When Freud discovered the truth he hoped and believed that his friend would die in six months. In fact Fleischl-Marxow's tortured body held out for six more years. The fundamentally flawed belief that cocaine could be used to treat morphine addicts persisted well into the 20th century.

Freud, of course, went on to greater things through his seminal work *The Interpretation Of Dreams*. His ideas formed the basis for psychoanalysis and, according to at least some Freud buffs, evolved because using cocaine allowed him to 'think outside the box'. What seems clear is that for 12 years, up until 1896, he was a regular user, even abuser, of cocaine.

BIRTH OF A GLOBAL BRAND

For a brief time, cocaine was viewed as a wonder drug – both by qualified doctors and the less-scrupulous quack-potions industry. It was certainly seized upon as a potential cure for morphine and opium use (a particularly serious problem in America where many Civil War veterans had returned to civvie street as junkies). An Atlanta pharmacist called John Pemberton was one of these addicts and in 1880 he decided to copy Mariani's idea of mixing coca with wine, producing his own uninspiringly named French Wine Coca. He marketed it as a general tonic and morphine substitute, and claimed it was regularly knocked back by 20,000 of the world's greatest scientists.

Things were looking good for Pemberton until 1885, when Atlanta's politicians banned all alcoholic drinks. Undeterred he went back to his laboratory and came up with a new concoction, mostly coca leaves and caffeine-rich kola nuts, sold through chemists as a concentrated syrup that buyers diluted with water or soda water. Pemberton needed a snappy trade name and by swapping the 'k' in kola for a 'c' he came up with something called Coca-Cola. Sounds vaguely familiar doesn't it?.

The drink didn't take off as Pemberton hoped and after six years he flogged the rights to an ex-medical student called Asa Griggs Candler for $2,300 (£1,600). It proved good business for Candler. When he took over, sales stood at 40,000 litres (9,000 gal) of syrup a year. Ten years later, at the turn of the century, he was shifting 1.7 million litres (370,877 gal) and, by the time he died in 1929, his personal fortune had topped $50 million (£34.5 million). Most of this success was achieved without the aid of cocaine, removed from the drink in 1905.

> In 1962 both Peru and Bolivia signed up to the Single Geneva Convention Against Drugs, agreeing to completely eradicate coca production in their countries within 25 years. Had this plan succeeded, in Peru alone it would have left 200,000 people out of work. Unsurprisingly, it didn't happen.

BAD MEDICINE?

Taking the coke out of Coke must have been a big commercial risk for Candler. The quack market had been awash with products such as Dr Don's Coca, Liebig's Coca Beef Tonic and Kumfort's Cola Extract. Because coca dried up the nasal passages it was mixed with snuff as a cure for hay fever and asthma – the first widespread use of sniffing to get a rush. You could buy wonderfully named preparations such as Dr Tucker's Specific or Anglo-

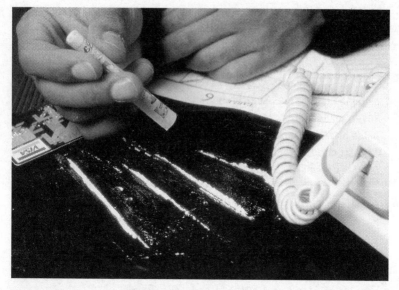

When snorted, cocaine is absorbed into the bloodstream through the nasal membrane, stimulating the central nervous system to produce feelings of alertness, exhilaration, and energy. Prolonged use of cocaine leads to anxiety, paranoia, psychological dependency, and damage to the lining of the nose (through snorting), while overdose can result in cardiac arrhythmia, seizure, and death.

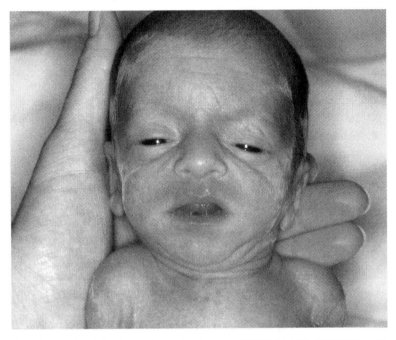

Face of a premature baby whose mother was a cocaine addict. Cocaine abuse may result in both a premature birth of and addiction in the unborn child. This tiny baby shows typical features of prematurity – it lacks subcutaneous fat, has a thin skin, and is covered with downy hair called *lanugo*. Apart from its immaturity, symptoms of which include immature internal organs, a pregnancy involving drug abuse may cause developmental abnormalities. In addition, this baby may suffer from cocaine withdrawal symptoms, for which it would have to be treated.

American Catarrh Powder. There were cough drops, toothache remedies, chewing 'paste' (the Inca never got proper credit for that one) and even coca cigarettes 'guaranteed to lift depression'. Cocaine could be bought from chemists as a neat solution or even as pure cocaine hydrochloride or 'powder coke'.

As the market expanded, so the price at first increased. Drugs companies such as Merck in Germany, and Parke, Davies of the USA, saw prices per gram quadruple soon after Koller's discovery to stand at $13 (£9). It couldn't last. More manufacturers flung themselves on to the bandwagon, there was oversupply and the price dropped. By the late 1880s, cocaine was so common that bar tenders were sprinkling it around liberally, what you might call Scotch with Attitude.

THE MAN WITH THE PLAN

The reason for the explosion in production was simple. In the past the big drugs companies had faced the same problem as the early medical researchers. They couldn't get enough coca leaf. It couldn't be grown in North America or western Europe and exporting bulky good-quality leaves was both expensive and difficult. Parke, Davies decided it needed a man in South America to check out possible new options. It chose Henry Hurd Rusby, recent medical graduate, botanist and, most importantly, a man with a brainwave.

Rusby reasoned that it must be possible to make cocaine on the spot. Trouble was, he didn't have a state-of-the-art pharmaceutical plant handy. He decided to improvize to see if there wasn't an easier, simpler way to produce the drug. The method he hit upon – still essentially the same used in the industry today – involved soaking the leaves in acid, shaking up the muddy brown result in alcohol to extract the alkaloids, adding an alkali like sodium bicarbonate, scooping out the dirty-white paste (known as *pasta basic*, or basic paste) and drying it out. The paste is up to two-thirds pure cocaine, it is compact and easy to transport, and is quickly converted into the final product: cocaine hydrochloride. In Peru, a new cocaine boom was born – 350 years after the Spanish one – in which processing factories as well as coca growers played a key role.

THE DOWNSIDE

Back at Coca-Cola, Candler wasn't so much worried by the competition as the fact that cocaine had side-effects. Side-effects were not good for business, particularly with the media homing in on a scandal. There had been a public relations disaster in 1902 when a court heard disturbing evidence that children were becoming addicted to the drink. Candler was having none of it and ordered cocaine to be removed from the Coke recipe. Meanwhile public unease was heightened by reports of hospital patients suffering from blackouts and convulsions and even dying as they received cocaine anaesthetics.

Health hazards were one thing, but when reports began to filter through of a link to violent crime, the Great American Public took a collective step backwards. The problem was that cocaine had become so easy to find that it was no longer the preserve of the filthy rich. People on limited incomes had got themselves habits they couldn't fund legally. What did they do? According to the government they robbed and stole to buy the drug, and they robbed and stole while they were high.

In March 1911 the head of America's anti-opium campaign, Dr Hamilton Wright, wrote to the *New York Times* expressing his concern: 'The misuse of cocaine is a direct incentive to crime ... It is perhaps of all factors a singular one in augmenting the criminal ranks. The illicit use of the drug is most difficult to cope with and the habitual use of it temporarily raises the power of the criminal to a point where, in resisting arrest, there is no hesitation to murder.'

This was bad enough. Next, some medical journals began reporting that 'the Negroes' in parts of the American south had become addicted to cocaine. Apparently many of them worked long shifts in the New Orleans docks and discovered that a sniff of that magic white powder they regularly unloaded allowed them to work longer and harder on less food. This was obviously fine with the dock management. Soon a vibrant drug market had sprung up, with local plantation workers also getting in on the act. By 1902 the *British Medical Journal* was telling how plantation owners had to issue cocaine rations to keep their men happy.

Three words to guarantee outrage in white, genteel America:

- blacks
- cocaine
- crime

Soon the newspapers were on the case with lurid reports of 'coke orgies', rapes and mass murders committed by blacks. One particularly ludicrous account was submitted by a police chief in Asheville, North Carolina, who told how a 'hitherto inoffensive Negro' had been driven mad by cocaine and pulled a knife. The officer placed his revolver over the man's heart and fired. He then fired a second shot into his chest. Neither of these bullets, claimed the cop, had any effect. The only thing that worked was to bludgeon that crazy Negro to death with a club. So he did and promptly headed off to buy a bigger gun.

Wow! So cocaine was making the 'goddamn Negroes' indestructible. Not only that, but when they had guns in their hands the drug turned them into formidable marksmen. In February 1914 the *New York Times* account of the above incident told how the 'cocaine nigger' had 'dropped five men dead in their tracks, using only one cartridge for each. The report adds that 'the deadly accuracy of the cocaine user has become axiomatic in Southern police circles'.

Not for the first time in the history of this drug – and all drugs – propaganda was accepted as fact.

KICKS FROM COCAINE …

At the end of the 19th century doctors, dentists and chemists accounted for a huge percentage of coke addicts. This was partly because they could get it easily, but they were also curious to check out its effects on themselves. There was a belief, held among some scientists even until the 1980s, that cocaine wasn't really addictive.

True, the early glut of production never developed into a national epidemic but this wasn't because the drug was benign. The reality is that new US laws were restricting availability – by 1922 dealers risked ten-year prison terms – and the street price was creeping up. Soon, ordinary American users couldn't *afford* to acquire a habit. Besides, as the 1930s dawned there were cheap new stimulants appearing, which were legal and, apparently, harmless. They were called amphetamines and their story is told elsewhere in this series.

The US cocaine market was perhaps ten years ahead of Europe's experience. Cocaine was still widespread in Paris (where half of all prostitutes were rumoured to be users), Barcelona, Madrid, Brussels, Berne and Rome. Germany, the world's biggest producer, had been ordered to cut back under the 1919 Treaty of Versailles, which ended World War I. The Germans had been stockpiling supplies, however, and in a country economically devastated by war these inevitably filtered on to the black market. People saw coke as a way to escape the national depression. Dealers cashed in, often eking out a stash by mixing in additional impurities.

> By the early 1980s an estimated 80 planes per night were making cocaine drops on Florida. Drug trafficking was thought to be the state's biggest earner and the coke sold topped $7 billion (£4.8 billion). This influx of wealth was reflected in property prices – 40 per cent of estates worth $300,000 (£200,000) or more were in foreign ownership.

In London, the *Daily Mail* reported that the drug was widely used among the West End's professional classes (barristers, politicians, actors and showbusiness types). Members of this young, smart and wealthy set were said to meet in designated flats or houses for 'a few doses of cocaine and a night of revelry'. Here was an early sign of the shifting cocaine culture. People began to see it as a drug of the upper classes and the 'gay young things' (that's gay in the traditional sense) of 1920s London. Cocaine was getting arty … and marching upmarket.

A KICK UP THE ARTS

Nowhere was this more obvious than in popular music and literature. One verse of the classic Cole Porter song 'I Get A Kick Out Of You' (covered in the 1980s by Roxy Music) opens with the words: 'I get no kick from cocaine'. After some subtle behind-the-scenes pressure – presumably to prevent apoplexy among conservatives – Porter's version was sometimes reworded 'Some get their perfume from Spain'. At least it rhymed.

There were plenty more examples of big-name singers and songwriters exploring cocaine themes. 'The Hop Song', later covered by Leadbelly, had originally included the following lines:

> *'Cocaine is for horses and not for men*
> *Doctors say it'll kill you but they don't tell you when*
> *Singing honey baby, honey baby, won't you be mine*
> *Take a sniff on me'*

The final line of a traditional blues song called 'Cocaine Lil' ran:

> *'They laid her out in her cocaine clothes*
> *She wore a snowbird hat with a crimson rose*
> *And on her tombstone you'll find this refrain*
> *She died as she lived, sniffing cocaine'*

And then there was the great 1930s blues classic 'Minnie The Moocher, which tells how the heroine 'fell in love with a guy named Smokey – she loved him though he was cokey'.

Fiction writers such as Agatha Christie and Dorothy Sayers both produced stories featuring cocaine addicts. Proust picks up the upper-class theme through his character the Vicomtesse de St Fiarcie, who destroys her good looks through overuse of the drug. The Russian-American novelist Vladimir Nabokov, whose best-known work was *Lolita*, once complained that his editor rejected a short story called 'A Matter Of Chance' on the basis that 'we don't print stories about cocainists'. But the biggest fictional coke addict of the age was none other than the world's greatest detective, that quintessential English hero Sherlock Holmes.

Holmes is first seen dabbling in the drug in *A Scandal In Bohemia*. Dr Watson tells how his friend alternates 'between cocaine and ambition', bizarrely attributing Holmes's drowsiness to his habit. This is probably because the author, Sir Arthur Conan Doyle, was not quite sure what cocaine actually does. He assumed that because it's an anaesthetic it must be a downer.

By the time Holmes confronts his dastardly adversary Moriarty in *The Final Problem*, Doyle has done his research. Holmes fans reading the adventures in order would have known that their hero was something of a coke-head because Watson tells how the detective once intravenously injected himself three times a day for three months; after which Doyle depicts the consequences of that abuse by giving Holmes classic symptoms of coke paranoia.

The Final Problem has the great man bursting into Watson's room, dashing around to close and fasten shutters, and warning of the dangers of airguns before ordering Watson to leave by the back garden wall rather than the front door. Then the irrational thoughts come tumbling out: Holmes talks of Moriarty as the 'author of half that is evil and nearly all that is undetected in this great city. He is a genius, a philosopher, and abstract thinker. He has a brain of the first order. He sits motionless, like a spider in the centre of its web, but that web has a thousand radiations, and he knows well every quiver of each of them.'

In his book *Cocaine: An Unauthorized Biography*, Dominic Streatfeild sets out the main arguments for Holmes's behaviour. One view is that because nobody but Holmes has ever seen Moriarty, the arch-criminal is a figment of the imagination – 'like an addict picking imaginary bugs from his skin, Holmes is plucking imaginary villains from his imagination', writes Streatfeild. An alternative explanation is that Moriarty is allegorical – the personification of cocaine or addiction itself. Whatever, Holmes does eventually emerge clean of the drug. In his final adventures we learn how he retires to an idyllic existence in Sussex to pursue hobbies of swimming and photography.

HIGH IN THE HILLS
Music? Literature? It could only be a matter of time before Hollywood also became a player in the cocaine trade. In the 1920s the emerging film industry with its pantheon of rich, hedonistic celebrities was a lucrative marketplace for cocaine dealers. Americans already perceived movie stars

as sex-and-drug crazed ne'er-do-wells and the Fatty Arbuckle scandal of September 1921, in which a young actress called Virginia Rappe died during a hotel party thrown by the silent screen comic, simply reinforced this view. In fact there was no proper evidence against Arbuckle, other than that he had consumed bootlegged drink in breach of Prohibition laws, but the popular press tried and sentenced him, and worked in a cocaine angle for good measure.

In fairness, making a link between Hollywood and cocaine was hardly wide of the mark. Arbuckle worked for Mack Sennett's Keystone Studios along with a young actress called Mabel Normand, who became embroiled in a high-profile murder case. She was ruined after being exposed as a cocaine addict with a truly awesome $2,000-a-month (£1,400) habit. Barbera La Marre, who starred alongside Douglas Fairbanks in his 1921 film *The Three Musketeers*, was said to keep a permanent stash of coke in her grand piano, using it to stay awake 22 hours a day (she later overdosed on heroin).

Good breeding made no difference. The acclaimed American actress Tallulah Bankhead, daughter of Democratic party leader and House of Representatives speaker William Brockman Bankhead, told in her autobiography how she once mistakenly put cocaine solution in her eyes, mistaking it for eyedrops. When a friend at the New York restaurant urged her to call a doctor, Bankhead threw a wobbly. 'I put the cocaine in my eyes and I don't tell that to doctors or anyone else,' she fumed. She is also, famously, the source of the quip 'Cocaine isn't habit-forming. I should know, I've been using it for years.'

In the eyes of middle-class America, Hollywood was built on 'happy dust' and booze. There was a clampdown by the police and a feeding frenzy among the press, resulting in a marked drop in use. Even so, some stars wouldn't leave cocaine alone. America's first 'drugs czar', Harry Anslinger, tells in his memoirs of the 'swashbuckling' actor who hawked himself around Europe trying to get the drug from doctors. This star – which only a blind Alaskan hermit would fail to recognize as Errol Flynn – claimed he needed the drug to cure everything from an inferiority complex to painful haemorrhoids. Flynn eventually admitted to Anslinger that he used cocaine to heighten sexual pleasure.

COCAINE GOES TO CUBA

By the end of World War II, cocaine had ceased to be a major problem in western society. It was still to be found in seedy London jazz clubs or Bohemian dinner parties but traditional smuggling routes had been so disrupted by war that in 1948 Anslinger found the drug in only one bust out of hundreds carried out. New laws restricted coca imports and confined legal cocaine manufacture to just two plants in New Jersey.

With such a dwindling market for coca leaves, Peruvian growers were staring bankruptcy in the face. Their own, legal, coke laboratories were forced out of business following a 1949 report by the United Nations Commission of Enquiry on the Coca Leaf. There was only one thing for it: to take production underground. This they did. Then they took their cocaine to Cuba.

The role of Cuba in worldwide cocaine smuggling is important for two reasons. First, because the violent, resourceful Cuban drugs gangs of the 1950s and 1960s effectively provided the model for the violent, resourceful Colombian drugs gangs of today. Second, because Cuba is the classic example of what happens when a major power uses sneaky tactics to undermine a government it doesn't like. In case you think this is just another piece of kick-the-meddling-Yanks polemic, I promise it isn't. All governments, of all political doctrines, do this and it's dead easy for commentators to stand back 40 years later and sadly shake their heads at the inevitable cock-ups. Even so, in the case of Cuba and cocaine, America really did cock up. Big time.

Why did the Peruvians go to Cuba in the first place? For one thing it was an ideal springboard into the American market. The coast of Florida lay barely an hour's flight away while Latin America was easily accessible for a bit of overland smuggling. There was also a ready market on the island. Ever since Fulgencio Batista took power in 1952, the US mob had controlled a millionaires' playground of late-night bars, clubs, strip joints and casinos. Holidaying Americans didn't know much about cocaine but they sure as hell liked it. Soon mobsters such as Meyer Lansky and Benjamin 'Bugsy' Siegel were expanding smuggling operations to include Chile, Mexico and Colombia. By the end of the 1950s, 90 per cent of the world's illegal cocaine was moved through Cuba.

Then a young communist revolutionary arrived to spoil the party. He was Fidel Castro and when he seized power in 1959 one of his first acts was to deport Lansky, Siegel *et al* back to the States. Soon waves of disgruntled anti-communist rebels – some of whom had made a buck or two from cocaine – were heading for Florida at the rate of 1,700 per week. The exiles wanted revenge on Castro. In America they found a willing ally in the form of the Central Intelligence Agency (CIA), which trained and equipped them as Brigade 2506. On 17 April 1961, about 1,300 of these rebels were landed in the Bay of Pigs, southern Cuba, intending to fight their way to Havana.

Cocaine trafficker Carlos Lehder set up base on Norman's Cay, a remote Bahamian island complete with airstrip, in 1977. Working with his partner George Jung his first flight to the United States carried 250kg (550lb), netting the pair a cool $1 million (£700,000). By 1980 Lehder was personally making $300 million (£200 million) a year.

It was one of the greatest and most embarrassing fiascos in the CIA's history. Within two days the Cuban army had killed 90 of the invaders and imprisoned the rest. President John F Kennedy was criticized by Republicans for failing to support the operation and by Democrats for allowing it to happen at all. The prisoners were gleefully put up for ransom by Castro and, eventually, most made it back to the States. But the damage was done. The remnants of Brigade 2506 were left to hang in the wind by the CIA, the only problem being that they didn't see it that way ...

Determined to try again they set about financing a private army. They knew about drugs trafficking and now (thanks to the CIA) they knew the techniques to avoid being caught. They made good money, some of which did indeed go towards attacking Castro's commies. Unfortunately an even larger slice of the profits found its way into the private accounts of individual leaders. As Florida's Cuban community grew, so did the number of drug barons' contacts. By the mid-1960s they were networking cocaine distribution across America.

Dominic Streatfeild sums up the problem this gave the Florida cops with a quote from a former Drugs Enforcement Agency (DEA) operative tasked with busting the Cubans.

'Who trained them? The CIA. And they trained them so goddamn well that in South Florida when you were doing a narcotics transaction one of the first things you looked for was counter-surveillance! They put out their own counter-surveillance! They weren't dummies. We trained them well.' One DEA bust in 1970 rounded up 150 Cubans. Seven in every ten were veterans of the Bay of Pigs shambles.

Throughout the 1960s and 1970s, the Cubans relied on Chilean cocaine factories. Then they reasoned that they could cut out the middleman by buying and processing their own coca. They asked the Colombians to help because they knew how successfully cartels there had sourced and sold both cocaine and marijuana. At roughly the same time the Chileans decided that *they* could improve margins by finding new distributors. Where did they go? You've seen this one coming. They went to Colombia.

COLOMBIA, COKE CENTRAL

Colombia had a long and lucrative tradition of smuggling, particularly luxury household goods, alcohol and precious stones. It was an undeveloped country with a long, remote coastline and easy access to the Panama Canal free trade area. No coca or cocaine had ever been produced there but, hey, so what? If it was valuable and you could smuggle it you could count the Colombian underworld in. Corruption was rife, drugs law enforcement negligible.

At first the Colombians simply set themselves up as middlemen, servicing both their Cuban and Chilean partners. Then they began to muscle in on their customers' territory, bidding for unrefined coca paste in Bolivia and Peru, cooking it up and distributing it across the USA. By 1970 the Colombian cartels had come from nowhere to challenge Cuban domination. Millions of young Americans revelling in the rebellion culture of the day decided cocaine was the new Big Thing; less dangerous than heroin or speed, more predictable than LSD, more exciting than marijuana and dead simple to take. Besides – and this was the clincher – it was supposed to take sexual orgasm to new heights.

Almost overnight – its image boosted by a plethora of rock songs and films such as *Easy Rider* – cocaine became easily accessible. *Rolling Stone* magazine declared it 'Drug of the Year' for 1970. *Newsweek* famously reported that 'orgasms go better with coke'. Students looking to make their fortunes worked out that you could buy a kilo (2¼lb) in Peru for $4,000 (£2,750), cut it, and sell it back home for $300,000 (£200,000). Oh, and in case there were any doubters one police narcotics chief told how cocaine produced 'a good high ... and you don't get hooked'. At San Francisco's Haight-Ashbury Free Clinic, Dr David Smith knew that this was untrue.

'Following the speed epidemic, heroin and cocaine really started hitting the US,' he recalls. 'Basically cocaine was then a white, middle-class type of drug. This was the '70s, people lived life in the fast lane and there was a general public perception that it was not addictive. This persisted even when we started to see users coming in with toxic symptoms and with cocaine psychosis. They were using it compulsively and they looked very much like the amphetamine abusers in terms of their addiction.

'We told anyone who would listen that cocaine acts like amphetamine, it is addictive if you use the broader definitions of addiction; it is highly toxic; it is very seductive and users will develop an upper-downer cycle. All of our predictions about its effects proved correct.'

THE DRUG LORDS OF COLOMBIA

The 1970s cocaine boom in America coincided with a major shift in production. Chile had always been a major supplier to the USA, but the coup by General Pinochet in 1973 was bad news for traffickers. Literally hundreds were rounded up and despatched on planes to America. It was Pinochet's way of saying thanks to the CIA for helping ease him into power.

Colombian drug barons moved quickly to full the vacuum. They had no shortage of muscle (the country was awash with guns after a civil war) and they were not afraid to use it – especially on foreigners and gringos trying their luck as cocaine smugglers. Soon any serious competition from American gangs was seen off, sometimes violently.

The leading cartels sent representatives to Bolivia and Peru to jack up coca production and ensure a steady supply. They bribed local cops and politicians to stop domestic interference. They also began sounding out Colombian nationals resident in America to see if anyone fancied making an easy buck as a distributor. The ex-pats usually did. Ever since Colombia's textile industry went belly-up in the 1960s there has been a steady stream of emigrants seeking a new life in the US of A. Unfortunately, that new life was uncannily similar to the old one – namely poverty and unemployment. For these people cocaine was a way out. They were well-placed to coordinate supply.

By the mid-1970s the minor players in Colombia had fallen by the wayside, often quite literally, courtesy of 100 rounds or so from a machine pistol. There was vicious fighting between the Colombians and the Cubans (the latter coming a distinct second) but DEA agents noted with interest that there was not always all-out war between the big cartels. On the contrary they sometimes struck alliances, combining shipments to share profits and swapping intelligence to guard against informers. The cities of Medellín and Cali became the centre of the cocaine business. Each had their own, notorious drug families.

In Cali, names in the frame included Helmer 'Pacho' Herrera, Jose Santacruz Londono and several members of the Rodriguez-Orejuela clan. In Medellín one of the first high-profile gangsters was a former prostitute called Griselda Blanco, aka the Black Widow (on account of her three husbands who had been killed in drug wars). Her other nicknames (you just can't be a proper gangster without them) included the Godmother, La Gaga (the Stutterer) and Muneca (Dollface).

GRISELDA BLANCO
In 1979 Blanco was the best-known – and most feared – cocaine trafficker in the United States. Then aged 36, she had transferred the hub of her operation to Miami. She was attractive, flamboyant and tried to work wherever possible with other women, especially widows. Drug folklore has it that she even designed her own knickers with hidden pockets suitable for carrying coke stashes through customs.

Her gang was known as Los Pistoleros and she had several hundred names on her payroll. These hitmen were credited with inventing a crude, but effective, assassination method in which a motorcycle driver and pillion passenger would draw alongside their target car in a busy city street. The pillion man would then empty his machine pistol into the occupants and the pair would high-tail it through traffic queues. But let it not be said that Blanco's killers were unimaginative. One was rumoured to tape shut the eyes and mouths of his victims, drain off their blood in the bath and neatly fold remaining skin and bone into old TV or hi-fi boxes.

Soon the DEA and the DAS (Colombia's equivalent of the FBI) were watching other major drug lords. There was Jorge Luis Ochoa Vasquez (the Fat Man), Jose Gonzalo Rodriguez Gacha (the Mexican), an underworld enforcer whose hobbies were – in order – violence, soccer (as in buying teams) and horses. There was the legendary Caribbean drug transporter known as Carlos Lehder. And then there was El Padrino (the Godfather), otherwise known as Pablo Escobar Gaviria. Together, these four were the brains behind the notorious Medellín cartel.

The DAS knew that rival traffickers would occasionally blow each other away, although they had no real conception of the term 'cocaine wars' until 22 November 1975 when air traffic controllers at Cali spotted a light plane trying to land under cover of the radar clutter surrounding an Avianca Airlines commercial flight. Police arrested the two pilots and recovered 600kg (1,320lbs) of cocaine – then the biggest seizure on record. There was mayhem on the streets, with 40 gangsters wiped out in a single weekend. Curiously, all the killings were in Medellín rather than Cali. Medellín was declared cocaine capital of the world.

EL PADRINO

The Medellín bosses were all ruthless, murdering, millionaire villains, but history will record Escobar (El Padrino – the Godfather) as the most successful. In fact he was arguably the greatest criminal the world has seen. Born into a middle-class background (his mother was a teacher and his father a farmer) he left high school with enough wit and intelligence to run a legitimate business. Instead he started work as a hi-fi smuggler's enforcer and graduated to kidnapping (a growth industry in 1970s Colombia).

When in 1976 he was arrested in possession of 39kg (86lb) of coke the DAS believed he was merely a drug 'mule' or delivery man. This view rapidly changed. First, Escobar's arrest order was mysteriously revoked.

Then the head of the DAS got a death threat. The two arresting cops were murdered along with their regional commander. The judge who ordered the arrest was murdered. A newspaper editor who wrote the story eight years later was murdered and his newspaper bombed. The moral of this tale? Don't bust Pablo Escobar Gaviria.

By the turn of the 1980s Escobar was wallowing in money. A cool $500,000 (£345,000) per day according to some estimates, rising to $1 million (£700,000) a day by the mid-1980s. These kind of sums are not easy to spend but Pablo did his best. He bought 2,800ha (7,000 acres) of land east of Medellín, built a luxurious ranch complete with swimming pools and, obviously, mortar emplacements, and hung a Piper Cub light airplane above the entrance gate. Everybody knew, especially the cops and drug agents, that this was the plane in which he had flown his first cocaine shipment to America.

Escobar didn't stop there. He bought dozens of wild animals, turned them loose in the ranch grounds and opened the place as a public zoo. He became Public Benefactor No.1 by building 500 houses in Medellín and giving them to poor families. He mended roads, built churches, wired in street lamps, paid for food wagons to tour poor estates and ensured that the residents got free private healthcare. Every year, at Christmas, he handed out 5,000 toys to underprivileged children. He even formed his own political party, called Civismo en Marcha (Good Citizenship on the March). In 1982 he got himself elected as a member of the Colombian parliament, a position that, under the constitution, guaranteed him immunity from prosecution.

In 1930 the cocaine market was hammered by the arrival of a new, legal stimulant called amphetamine. New York City records show that, whereas there were 239 coke-linked convictions between 1921 and 1925, the total number of coke users sentenced over the following four years was just 27.

JORGE OCHOA

That same year Colombia was reeling under a new threat from a revolutionary Marxist group calling itself M-19. It was raising cash for the cause through kidnapping and on 12 November 1981 its terrorists abducted Marta Nieves Ochoa from outside Medellín's Antioquia University. This was a bad mistake. It was one thing to target industrialists and politicians. It was quite another to lift one of the five Ochoa sisters. Jorge Ochoa was suitably unimpressed and, within a couple of weeks, a summit of all the major drug cartels had formed a vigilante group known as Muerte a Secuestradores (Death to Kidnappers).

Three weeks after Marta's kidnap, a light airplane banked gently over a crowded football stadium in Cali and dropped some leaflets announcing that 233 'businessmen' had formed the MAS to stamp out kidnapping. The wording of the leaflet suggested that Jorge and his mates weren't messing about: 'The basic objective will be the public and immediate execution of all those involved in kidnappings beginning from the date of this communiqué ... [they] will be hung from the trees in public parks or shot and marked with the sign of our group – MAS.'

The statement warned that jailed kidnappers would be murdered or, if this proved impossible, 'retribution will fall on their comrades in jail and on their closest family members'.

Within six weeks 100 M-19 members had been captured and handed over to the police. No one knows precisely how many were murdered, but judging by the speed with which Marta was freed, M-19 was clearly anxious to end this little spat. The word on the street was that the Ochoa family never did pay the $12 million (£8.3 million) ransom.

It looked as though Escobar, Jorge Ochoa *et al* were the unofficial rulers of Colombia. With their private armies and huge resources they feared no one. Occasionally there was an inter-gang feud but nothing they couldn't handle. As for the government, its efforts at drug control were barely even irritating.

ENTER THE ENFORCERS

Until, that is, in August 1983 when newly elected president Belisario Betancur appointed a determined young congressman called Lara Bonilla as his Minister of Justice. Bonilla recognized that drug money was destroying his country's economy because it required a vast black market to prosper.

He began by asking awkward questions; how did Colombia's mega-millionaires make their money? Why did they need all those aeroplanes? Escobar's people tried bribes to keep him quiet, then death threats. But it made no difference; Bonilla publicly branded Escobar a trafficker and ordered his chief of police Jaime Ramirez to bust every cocaine laboratory in the country.

Ramirez was a rare jewel in Colombian law enforcement circles. He was incorruptible. So when in 1984 he was informed by the DEA of a major cocaine plant deep in the Colombian jungle he organized an attack so secret that none of the police and army officers knew where they were going until they were actually in the air.

The DEA's intelligence was spot on, not least because their undercover people had sold a huge consignment of anhydrous ethyl ether – a key ingredient of the cocaine production process – to a Medellín cartel representative called Frank Torres. In with the ether barrels were some satellite beacons, and soon the DEA was analyzing satellite photos of a 1km (0.6 mile) airstrip in the middle of nowhere. The photos didn't need much analysis. Neither did the amount of radio traffic beaming out of the place.

The lab was called Tranquilandia and once the Colombian SWAT team had seen off its guards they knew they had hit the motherlode. It looked like something from a James Bond set: a huge complex with quarters for guards, chemists, pilots and cooks; there were hot showers, flushing toilets, mains electricity and weapons stores; and everywhere lay thousands upon thousands of chemical drums. One logbook showed the place had processed 15 tonnes/tons of cocaine paste in January and February that year.

Ramirez's men also found a pilot's notebook containing a convenient map of labs in the area with radio frequencies. Over the next few days the raiders visited each of them: Cocolandia, where a tonne/ton of the drug was wrapped in waterproof packaging; Cocolandia 2 (500kg/1,100lb); Tranquilandia 2 (4 tonnes/tons); El Diamante (half a tonne/ton). Over the next fortnight Ramirez recovered 8,500kg (18,700lb) of pure cocaine and 1,500kg (3,300lb) of cocaine base. He seized seven planes, nine labs and 12,000 chemical drums. The whole shooting match was worth over $1 billion (£0.7 billion). Even by Medellín standards this was serious spondulicks.

Lara Bonilla rightly took the credit for the operation. He also knew he was a dead man walking. He told a journalist friend that he would be killed on 30 April 1984 and, sure enough, that afternoon two young hitmen hired by the cartel roared alongside his official car on a Yamaha motorbike – in classic Los Pistoleros style – and sprayed the back seat with bullets. Lara's bodyguards opened up immediately, killing one and injuring the other. But it was too late. Colombia had lost the one man truly capable of striking back at the drug lords.

President Betancur responded in a national radio broadcast at 3am the following morning. He described the drugs business as the most serious problem in Colombian history and pledged a 'war without quarter' against traffickers. Escobar and his friends weren't unduly worried. They'd heard this kind of stuff before. But Bonilla's memorial service wiped the smiles off their faces. During his address Betancur announced that: 'Colombia will hand over criminals wanted in other countries so that they may be punished as an example.' He got a standing ovation from the congregation.

> Leaders of the Medellín cartel made an extraordinary truce offer to Colombia's President Betancur in 1984: they would dismantle their trafficking networks, ending three-quarters of the country's cocaine output, provided that they could keep the $2 billion (£1.4 billion) they'd already made. Betancur turned them down after news of the talks leaked out.

Reintroducing extradition was a brave move. Escobar, Ochoa and their lieutenants knew that if ever they got hauled before an American court they would never taste freedom again. Bribes and escape plots would be useless. So, like Betancur, the Medellín cartel also prepared for war without quarter. The result was an unprecedented level of bombings and killings on the streets, an increasing cycle of violence in which American diplomats, DEA officers and their families also became prime targets.

The country was now quite literally a war zone. At one point, anti-tank rockets were fired at the US Embassy and government tanks were deployed to end an M-19 terrorist siege at Bogotá's Palace of Justice. Almost 150 people died in the subsequent shoot-out. Judges, journalists and their families were threatened or murdered, and in 1986 the main cause of death for adult males in Colombia was not heart disease or cancer but murder. Shootings in Medellín alone were reported at an average of almost ten per day. In 1988 and 1989 it is estimated that death squads accounted for 40,000 citizens. And amid all this death and destruction, the Medellín and Cali cartels began fighting a turf war.

For the Colombian government the killing was too high a price. Extradition had to end. In 1990, after an election campaign in which three presidential candidates were murdered, Liberal Party leader César Gaviria Trujillo, was elected. Two months later his new constitution banned the extradition of Colombian citizens and Gaviria offered an amnesty to drug traffickers who turned themselves in. Pablo Escobar was among those who obliged.

He was sent to prison to await trial. But it was a funny kind of prison because, well, Pablo owned it. There was a health club, a marijuana plot, a disco, a motorbike scrambling track, chalets for entertaining women visitors – even an underground bomb-proof bunker. The prison 'cells' all had videos, TVs and hi-fis. Escobar had the telephones and fax lines he needed to run his business, and enjoyed the occasional trip to a soccer match – under police escort, of course. It was all quite hunky-dory, until he got too cocksure.

Perhaps to emphasize that he was still in charge, Escobar tortured and killed two former associates who had been trying to negotiate a reduction on the monthly $1 million (£700,000) 'tax' he'd levied on their cocaine trafficking. The police decided this was too much. Pablo should go to a proper prison. Inevitably, though, he was tipped off and in July 1992 simply discharged himself. He went into hiding in the heart of Medellín, moving from house to house and communicating from moving cars to prevent his phone calls being traced.

Had he not ordered those last two gangland killings he might have pulled it off. But now even Pablo's own people feared he was going insane. They wondered if he would turn on them next and some key aides defected to the Cali cartel – then headed by Pacho Herrera and the Rodriguez Orejuela brothers – for protection. Now Escobar had not only the DAS, DEA and CIA after him but a new organization called Los PEPES (People Persecuted by Pablo Escobar). It was run by the Cali boys.

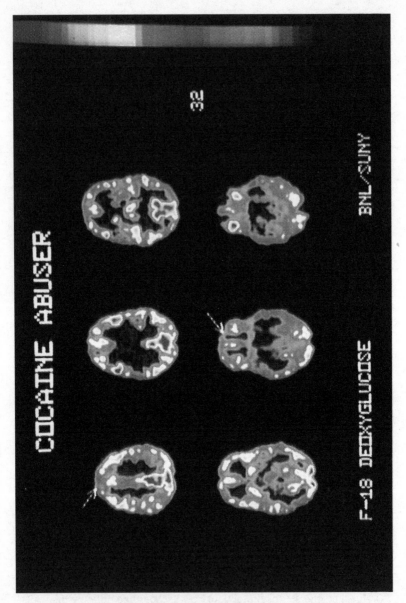

PET (Positron Emission Tomography) scans showing the brain a cocaine user. The front of the brain is at the TOP, and the slices get deeper from LEFT-RIGHT. The shaded bar (RIGHT) shows decreasing activity from light to dark. A cocaine user's brain is less active than a healthy brain — the arrows show the area of the frontal lobes, where activity is markedly lower.

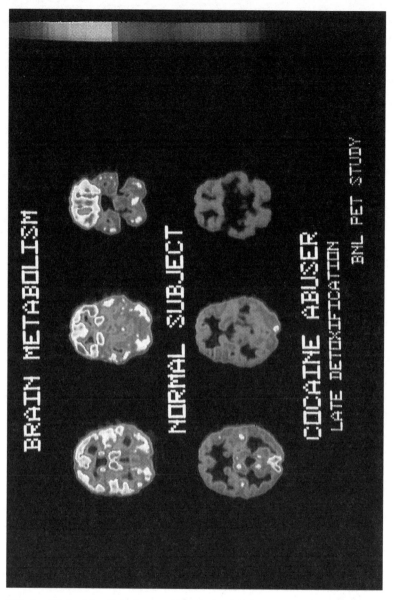

PET scan of horizontal sections of a normal brain (TOP) and the brain of a cocaine user after four months of abstinence (BOTTOM), with the brighter shapes indicating areas of high activity. The brain of the cocaine user is shown to be less active than the healthy brain, even after four months without the drug.

By November police mobile tracking units had pinpointed Escobar's phone calls to a 200 sq m (2000 sq ft) area of the city. It was far too densely populated to surround, so they played a waiting game hoping his guard would slip. On 2 December it did. He stayed put rather than talk on the move and he spoke for six minutes, long enough to get a secure signal fix. Then he was seen at a window and commando-trained police moved in. Pablo was not the kind of guy to be taken alive. And he wasn't.

Escobar is now a distant memory, yet for Colombia's new cocaine kings the past decade has been business as usual. When you hear politicians talk of the 'war on drugs' they usually forget to mention that it's a war that patently isn't being won. Certainly not by destroying coca fields or raiding traffickers. Not by prosecuting dodgy chemical manufacturers and money launderers. Not by busting backstreet labs and dealers. Deep down, law enforcement agencies know and privately accept this. The cocaine trade abhors a vacuum and there'll always be someone willing to blow in and make a fortune. In reality, all the cops can do is make life tough for the bad guys.

Cocaine will always be in circulation. The question is, will it be in your circulation?

'The biggest high from your brain's neurotransmitters is meant to be sex. That's your orgasm. When you are taking cocaine you are leap-frogging way over that.'

– Aidan Gray, national coordinator, COCA

COCAINE, SEX AND THE FEEL-GOOD FACTOR

So why try cocaine in the first place? That's easy. Because it's there. You don't need a degree in psychology to know that experiments are part of being young, part of life. If our brains didn't encourage us to experiment, evolution would be hard work.

Hold on, you say, if that's right, how come we're not all doing coke. Same reason we're not all doing kung-fu or economics degrees. Cocaine is not a part of every peer group and millions will go through life never seeing it close up. Some of us will walk away after weighing up the health risks. Some will think sniffing powder is too disgusting. Some will think it's too expensive. Some will stick to collecting bottle tops. But some will give it a try and like it.

There's nothing shameful about liking recreational drugs. Most of us do – that's why the drinks, tobacco and coffee industries make such big bucks. The danger really lies in how much we like them and on this count cocaine knocks every other mind-manipulating substance into a cocked hat. The reason lies in the unique way it works on the brain.

If you've ever had a sexual orgasm you'll know how wonderful it feels. That's because your unconscious brain regards the reproductive act as the single most important thing you can do with your life. Forget global warming, democracy, human rights, scientific discovery, justice, racial equality and all the other great issues of the day. As far as your brain is concerned, pal, your number one duty is to get laid.

Unless, of course, you are a regular cocaine user.

BETTER THAN SEX …
Dr Bill Jacobs, assistant professor of addiction medicine at Florida University's Department of Psychiatry, explains it like this: 'When you take cocaine you create an artificial stimulus to your brain's reward pathway. The pathway is there to keep our species alive – it's food, water, nurturing the young and especially sex. These are all natural rewards which turn on the reward pathways and tell us: "You did good, do that again."

'If those natural rewards turn on the pathway to a value of one, well, cocaine turns it on to a value of 1,000. That is just not a natural phenomenon. Our brains are not made to run like that. When you remove the cocaine you immediately start to fall from a much higher place.'

Aidan Gray, national coordinator for the UK charity Conference on Crack and Cocaine (COCA), describes the buzz in more colloquial terms. The former drug project worker has specialized in cocaine since 1994 and is among Europe's leading authorities on its effects. He seemed like a good person to ask about comparisons between cocaine and sex, because those comparisons certainly exist. Cocaine's reputation as an aphrodisiac dates back almost to the time it was first produced.

'I came across women who would have unprotected sex for rocks of crack,' he recalls. 'We're not talking about prostitutes. These were ordinary women who wouldn't buy crack themselves but would have casual sex with a crack-smoking partner, maybe someone who would bring it round to their house. The attraction of this arrangement was usually that home was a safe place to smoke.

'Is cocaine an aphrodisiac? I'm not sure that's the right word. It certainly does increase anticipation and if you've ever been to a theme park like Disneyland and you're waiting for the big ride you'll know that sense of "Ohmigod! What am I doing?" That's your fight or flight response. It's where craving comes from. It's your heart beating, the funny churning in your stomach, the sweating – all that stuff. It is rooted in anticipation.

Like at school when you have a first date with someone you really fancy, there's that strange giddy feeling. Anticipation and sex are very closely linked.

'The other connection is the brain's pleasure-giving neurotransmitters. There's a definite tick alongside cocaine's effect on dopamine and a lot of scientists think seratonin is also a factor. Cocaine works on reward. When you have lunch and you enjoy it you get a small release of neuro-transmitters and that reinforces your behaviour. Your brain knows that eating is good for you.

Injecting cocaine vastly increases a person's chances of contracting hepatitis C. Estimates suggest that between 65 per cent and 90 per cent of needle users become infected. National Institute on Drug Abuse research report, May 1999

'The biggest high from your brain's neurotransmitters is meant to be sex. That's your orgasm. When you are taking cocaine you are leap-frogging way over that. The brain mechanisms are very similar for sex and coke. So when you combine a sexual partner, a gram or two and perhaps a bottle of champagne you can see why people think there is an aphrodisiac effect. The pleasure is both physical and neurological.

'In the long run, however, this pleasure diminishes. Women I've worked with tend to say "Actually, I'd rather just have the cocaine." They'll use sex as a way to get the cocaine but it is not their main motive. With men it's kind of like well, the mind is willing but the flesh is weak. Gradually, cocaine becomes the precise opposite of an aphrodisiac. It is more pleasurable than sex and so it becomes the preferred option.

'I've known plenty of users who like smoking a crack pipe while they watch others have sex. Some prefer a porn video. Still others want a blow job – especially if they can't achieve a full erection. There is a sexual connection but it doesn't affect everybody and it isn't the same thing as an aphrodisiac.

'One dangerous practice is the use of cocaine and Viagra [the impotency drug] together. The obvious conclusion is that it must be a brilliant cocktail because there's the sexual anticipation you get from coke and the ability to have repeated sex from Viagra.

'The trouble is that the warning labels on the Viagra box all involve cardiovascular problems. When you take cocaine or crack it increases the amount of endophilin in your body to three or four times normal levels. This is a chemical that constricts your blood vessels. So the cocaine is increasing your heart rate and blood pressure but there is less space for the blood to get through. It's like putting your thumb over the end of a hose. It is not a good idea.'

Dopamine, seratonin – let's face it, these aren't names to concentrate your mind as you snort a line or achieve sexual ecstasy (unless you are an unbelievably sad person). But neurotransmitters seem to be at the core of cocaine addiction, and the reason why taking the drug is so much fun. Thanks to scientists such as Dr Nora Volkow we now know a lot more about them.

ALL IN THE MIND?
During studies at the University of Texas, Houston, in 1984 Volkow noticed that the brains of cocaine users showed severe changes. She began photographing them using a positron emission tomography scanner - a process that involves tagging molecules with radioactive particles (positrons), injecting them into the blood and monitoring their voyage around the brain. She quickly discovered that cocaine has a special relationship with neurotransmitters such as dopamine.

First, what's a neurotransmitter? Imagine the wiring in your house. You switch on a light and because this completes an electrical circuit, the bulb is powered into life. Your brain also uses electrical circuits but it doesn't mess about with cumbersome physical connections. Instead it completes circuits by sending chemicals – neurotransmitters – from one nerve cell to another. This happens almost instantaneously. Neurotransmitters make your body perform physical functions – talking, sneezing, cutting toenails – but they also handle emotion and instinct for survival. Eating chocolate, taking a hot shower, drinking ice-cold beer in a heatwave, cuddling your kids and (especially) having sex – dopamine makes all these experiences feel good for various evolutionary reasons.

Dopamine messengers are being released into synapses (the spaces between nerve cells) all the time. But they don't hang around because your brain immediately sends out transporters to round them up and shepherd them back to their cells ready for next time. This is called re-uptake. If it didn't happen, your orgasm would last all afternoon and disturb your post-coital nap.

Cocaine uses sneaky tactics to disrupt this mechanism. It attaches itself to perhaps two-thirds of your dopamine transporters and disables them. The stranded dopamine keeps swirling around the spaces, or synapses, between nerve cells and does its genetic duty by dispensing euphoric joy. That's your cocaine high and it will last for between 40 and 60 minutes, depending on the method of consumption.

What happens then is unpleasant. After attaching itself to a dopamine transporter the cocaine detaches fairly quickly (although traces remain in the brain for two to three days). If no more arrives the dopamine is duly rounded up, except now the process becomes much more rigorous. It's as though the brain is a fussy mother, angry that her kids have been out too long. Dopamine levels fall below normal – below the level they existed prior to cocaine intake – and, sure enough, that's your crash. The immediate urge is to take more cocaine, to 'binge' until either supplies run out or exhaustion takes over.

All this happens within your medial forebrain bundle, the structures of which are your frontal cortex, nucleus accumbens and ventral tegmental area. Most recent research has focused on what happens when dopamine leaves the ventral tegmental area and heads for the nucleus accumbens. In this area of the brain lie the roots of addiction. Scientists can argue about whether it's a physical or psychological addiction, but addiction it is. When you take cocaine regularly your brain physically alters.

The most obvious change is a drop in the number of dopamine receptors on nerve cells. With fewer receptors, those nerves are denied normal levels of stimulation and so pleasurable experiences other than cocaine no longer induce familiar feelings of 'natural' happiness. This is why some of Aidan Gray's clients preferred coke to sex.

For reasons not fully understood it seems that taking cocaine irregularly may sensitize some people (they become more responsive to the same dose). But regular use leads to tolerance and so more of the drug is needed to reach the same level as a previous high. Evidence suggests that, for regular users, dopamine receptors become permanently damaged and the brain never manages to restore them to pre-cocaine levels. This creates a huge problem for those seeking treatment because their desire for the drug is never quite diminished. They remember it as the only thing that delivered true pleasure. The best they can hope for is to resist their craving until enough dopamine receptors come back into play, allowing other things in life to feel pleasurable again.

According to Dr Volkow the bingeing tendency may be caused by cocaine's ability to dabble in other areas of the brain, specifically the bits that tell us when we've had enough. This is our 'satiety' response. Volkow believes that in switching it off, cocaine ensures that users binge even though they know they will suffer at the end of it.

'Pleasure is a natural reinforcer to increase the probability that a species will engage in a given behaviour and continue that behaviour,' she told a National Institute on Drug Abuse research briefing in July 1998. 'Once these urges have been satisfied the body's normal response is satiety or "that's enough". When satiety is suppressed, the pleasurable properties of cocaine serve as a trigger for activating brain pathways that will then maintain the drug-consuming behaviour.'

Cocaine experiments on animals support this view, even though the behaviour of caged creatures is unlikely to mirror that of free human beings. In the 1960s researchers gave one group of laboratory rats unlimited access to heroin while another group got unlimited coke. Heroin is a sedative or 'downer' and so these rats tended to sleep more. Their consumption became routine and regulated. The cocaine rats on the other hand didn't stop self-administering hits until they became physically exhausted. They didn't sleep or eat and after waking from a collapsed state they immediately took more of the drug. They were all dead inside a month. The heroin rats by this time had developed a habit yet groomed, slept and ate fairly normally.

There are plenty more examples of animal experiments that

> The average age at which heart attacks are experienced by cocaine users is 44, compared to 61 in the general population.
> London *Guardian*, 10 August 1999

demonstrate cocaine's extraordinary power over brain function. In one case a chimp was trained to hit a bar to receive a single dose of coke. Once he'd worked this out, researchers began increasing the number of times he needed to hit the bar to get the same dose. The aim was to measure the addictive potential of the drug and scientists assumed there would come a point where the chimp had to press the bar so many times for his fix that he'd get bored and find something else to do. He didn't. They stopped the experiment after he pressed the bar 12,800 times for a single shot – 100–1,600 per cent more than for any other drug.

HARD HABIT TO BREAK

One of the more persistent 'media myths' is that crack cocaine hooks you instantly. But is it a myth? According to scientists at the Ernest Gallo Clinic and Research Centre in San Francisco, part of the University of California, a single coke dose can trigger a surge of activity among dopamine-sensitive brain cells. Experiments (*Nature*, May 2001) showed that mice were sensitized to cocaine after first exposure. In effect their dopamine cells became twice as responsive. Dr Antonello Bonci, senior author of the research paper and assistant professor of neurology at the university, said the study showed how cocaine strengthened connections between the nerve cells responsible for learning and memory. 'The single exposure appears to hijack the brain's normal molecular mechanisms of memory formation for about a week,' he said. His colleague, Dr Mark Ungless, went even further. 'What's so amazing is that nearly all dopamine neurons [nerve cells] are affected by this single cocaine exposure,' he said. 'This kind of response is rare and would have a profound effect throughout the brain – particularly other areas involved in addiction.'

The results of experiments with cocaine-taking macaque monkeys, published in February 2002, are equally intriguing. A team led by Professor Michael Nader at America's Wake Forest University divided the monkeys into small social groups and gave them open access to cocaine. The animals' brains were scanned for dopamine activity, and the social pecking order of the groups was monitored.

The scientists discovered, against expectations, that the dominant macaques had higher dopamine counts (making them happier) than their subordinates. More remarkably, these dominant individuals didn't simply hog the cocaine bar to keep the goodies for themselves. Rather, they used less cocaine and adopted a steady intake. It was in the lower echelons of the group that bigger and bigger fixes were needed.

There is an irresistible human comparison to draw here. Among wealthy and powerful members of society – say Wall Street executives and Bundestag politicians – cocaine use can be 'managed' to avoid lifestyle disruption. Yet in the squats and ghettos, regular users quickly descend into the abyss of addiction.

This is obviously over-simplistic but most scientists already accept that our addiction 'switch' depends on a blend of biology, psychology and disposable income. Comparatively few snorters end up as hopeless cases. In fact, everything about powder coke culture suggests that most people can, and do, regulate intake without a problem. So why all the fuss about crack cocaine. If it's essentially the same drug it must have the same health effects and consequences. This is an entirely reasonable conclusion. It's also completely wrong.

WHAT'S THE CRACK?

Ever wondered why you can't get hooked on nicotine quit-smoking patches? Why no one ever pleads with their neighbourhood pharmacist for 'just one more patch' to get through the day. After all, this is the same drug smoked by billions; the drug that is so seductive when inhaled. A patch contains as much as a few cigarettes. How come nicotine hooks you one way but not the other?

It's simple. The reason people like recreational drugs is that they crank up the pleasure centre of the brain. The more drugs you take the greater the pleasure rush, at least up to the point where you overdose. But, more importantly, it's the speed with which these drugs hit the brain that really counts. If you inhale them they go straight into your main blood vessels and you're in the fast lane to Pleasure City. If you snort, drink, eat or 'patch' them, then they have to trog around the back roads of your circulatory system before they find the freeway. The eventual rush will be more gradual and less intense, although it'll last longer.

This is the essential difference between a patch and a cigarette. It's also the difference between snorting powder coke and smoking crack cocaine. Because the high is more intense there's a powerful incentive to light up again as soon as the (equally intense) crash takes over. But before we tell the story of crack we need to know more about its parentage. That means a trip back to the 1970s and the amazing new wonder drug of America's *Easy Rider* generation. Cocaine freebase.

FANCY FREEBASE?

When you sniff cocaine you're actually consuming cocaine hydrochloride (or cocaine salt). The production process for this has essentially remained the same since a young student called Albert Niemann discovered it while working at the University of Gottingen in 1859. Niemann washed coca leaves in alcohol and sulphuric acid, distilled off the alcohol and separated out a resin, which he shook with bicarbonate of soda. This substance was again distilled to produce the now familiar, rod-shaped white crystals.

A quarter of a century later, drugs companies discovered a simpler method, which could be carried out on-site in South America's coca plantations (avoiding the problems associated with exporting fast-rotting coca leaves). They dowsed leaves in acid, shook up the sludgy result with alcohol, added a strong alkali such as bicarbonate of soda and, hey presto!, basic paste or *pasta basica*. This is between 40 and 65 per cent pure and is still the form most favoured by traffickers. It is a rough mixture of contaminated cocaine compounds, which is designed to be further refined into cocaine hydrochloride higher up the trading chain. As paste it can be smoked because it vaporizes quickly when heated. Ordinary powder coke just degrades. Light it and you might as well burn money.

Now the freebase story gets a tad speculative and confusing. According to the world's leading authority on the history of cocaine science, the University of California's Professor Ron Siegel, here's what probably happened.

Around 1970 a pioneering American cocaine trafficker in Peru notices production workers puffing away at something they call base. He tries it, likes it and, back in the USA, he smokes a bit of his usual cocaine hydrochloride mixed with tobacco. But something is wrong. There's no big rush. So he calls a friend with some chemistry know-how and asks why base might be different. They check out a textbook and discover the definition of a chemical 'base'.

They establish that cocaine hydrochloride (cocaine salt) can easily be converted back to base form by removing the hydrochloride molecule. This involves adding a strong alkali and dissolving everything in a solvent, such as ether. The ether stage is a bit dodgy because the fumes ignite so easily, but once the cocaine dries and crystallizes out it's in a stable form ready for smoking. The amateur chemists call this 'freeing the base' or freebasing.

Their one error is to assume that what the Indians call base and what their textbook calls base are one and the same. Not so. What they end up smoking is close to pure cocaine, not some mish-mash of coke-plus-impurities. In drinking terms it's the difference between a light beer and a similar quantity of 90 per cent proof Polish vodka. In other words, completely different.

Cooking freebase was a big secret at first. You needed high-quality cocaine (not easy to come by in the early 1970s), a mini chemistry lab – with beakers, measuring jars and solvents – and a decent understanding of the process. The presence of a fire extinguisher was also advisable, as Richard Pryor discovered. Those in the know would hire themselves out at parties, jealously guarding the secrets of their trade. Because it was a secret, everybody quickly worked it out. Siegel estimates that, by 1980, 300,000 freebase kits had been sold across America.

By then, users and scientists alike had realised that freebase was a new phenomenon. Smokers developed bizarre traits, such as constantly staring at the floor searching for a mislaid bit of base. When sharing a pipe they would bicker like children over sweets. Siegel's book *Intoxication* tells how he usually had to provide lab monkeys with a reward to persuade them to smoke drugs. With freebase they needed no reward. One monkey would even try to lick the smoke she exhaled. When Siegel conducted tests on men who had never smoked freebase they spontaneously ejaculated, even though their penises were flaccid. Euphoria was being redefined.

Some cocaine dealers, such as the notorious Ricky Ross – aka Freeway Rick – of South Central, Los Angeles, began offering clients prepared freebase to save them the trouble of cooking up powder coke. Because freebase comes in chunks, and because Ross had natural marketing flair, he called his product Ready Rock. When demand went ballistic he bought and converted houses into fully equipped freebase factories. In 1982 he was processing 15kg (33lb) per week. Two years later production hit 50kg (110lb) per week. As his buying power increased, so the price plummeted – from $25,000 (£17,250) down to a low of $9,500 (£6,500) per kilo (2¼lb). From being an expensive, white middle-class kind of drug, freebase was suddenly available to poorer Hispanic and black communities. At his peak, Ross cleared profits of $100,000 (£70,000) a day.

> Andean Indians believe that coca relieves hunger, reduces fatigue and promotes warmth. 'This belief is so strong that they may refuse to perform normal labour without it and in fact consume more coca during the cold season. 'Use Of Coca Leaf In Southern Peru', Hanna and Hornick

As the Los Angeles Times reported on 20 December 1994, 'If there was an eye of the storm, if there was a criminal mastermind ... if there was one outlaw capitalist most responsible for flooding LA's streets with mass-marketed cocaine, his name was Freeway Rick.'

There was another factor, though, for which Ross couldn't take the rap. As more people became familiar with freebase so they experimented with new ways to prepare it. Soon cooks discovered a method that avoided fiddling with beakers and dodging ether fireballs. They just heated ordinary coke powder in a solution with baking soda until the water evaporated. Dead easy. When this type of freebase was lit and smoked it made a crackling sound. If you were a drug dealer what street name would you have come up with?

AMERICA GETS CRACKING

On 17 November 1985, the New York Times told the world: 'Three teenagers have sought treatment already this year ... for cocaine dependence resulting from the use of a new form of the drug called "crack", or rock-like pieces of prepared freebase.' The media descended like vultures. Rightly or wrongly, 'crack' became the hyped-up horror story of the 1980s.

Over at the Haight-Ashbury Free Clinic, Dr David Smith had seen it all coming. 'We have a long history with cocaine,' he said. 'It's not a simple story. At HAFC we started out dealing mainly with bad acid [LSD] trips – these were young people from around the country who had a make-love-not-war-turn-on-tune-in-drop-out attitude. Whatever you think of them, at least they had a philosophy. At that time I was studying psychedelic drugs, amphetamines and the mechanisms of action. I knew that amphetamine acted in the brain in the same way as cocaine, they're both psycho-stimulants.

'The establishment didn't want to fund us so we built the clinic on rock'n'roll. Janis Joplin did benefits for us, Jefferson Airplane, The Grateful Dead, Carlos Santana – many big names came to help get us up and running. There was a something of a speed [amphetamine] culture around here. It was big in the western part of the US at that time and it moved east very quickly. We saw a huge increase in violence and in 1968 I saw for the first time what I call the "three Cs" of addiction – compulsion, loss of control and continued use despite adverse consequences.

'Then you had the arrival of crack cocaine. In medicine and pharmacology you teach by group – you don't view every drug as different. I would tell students that crack cocaine was very toxic, very addictive – just like amphetamine. But its preparation helped dictate some of the cultural components. We started seeing crack cocaine on the east coast while we were still dealing with amphetamine over here in the west. There was a paper published in the *Journal Of Psychoactive Drugs* about coca paste, a crude form of cocaine. This paste was really the forerunner of crack cocaine. It was pre-prepared for ease of handling, and much less expensive.

'When you snort cocaine you are actually snorting cocaine hydrochloride. With freebase you have an extraction process in which you "basefy" the drug – that is, you extract the hydrochloride using an organic solvent and you dry it. This lowers the vaporization point. When people talk about smoking cocaine what they really mean is vaporizing it. When you freebase, you heat the drug, vaporize it, inhale and you get a blood and brain level similar to an injection.

'With crack it's all pre-prepared. You don't extract it yourself or do any of that. The supplier mixes it with baking soda, which is the base, puts it in the microwave and then cracks off pieces – they call them rocks – to sell. That's one explanation for the drug's name. The other is that it crackles when you smoke it. Either way, it's the fast food of drug culture.

'The analogy I use sounds very simplistic but it gets the message through. Freebase is like a barbecue party. You have your barbecue pit and you go get a bun and a burger, you get all your condiments lined up and all your cooking utensils, and away you go. That's the kind of ritual the middle and upper classes follow.

'Crack cocaine is like going out for a McDonald's takeaway burger. It costs a lot less and it's all pre-prepared. We saw the crack cocaine epidemic explode and it moved immediately into the lower socio-economic non-white populations. It was no longer a drug of the white middle class but of the lower-class black culture.

'With crack you buy a rock for $20 (£14) and away you go. It's a street drug and you can easily carry it around. With freebase you've got to have all the equipment – which means paying out around $100 (£70) – and it requires a lot more skill. You have to be careful that you don't produce something that will make you lose perspective and burn yourself up like Richard Pryor.

'I treat a lot of crack cocaine addicts and when you ask how much they are taking they will always talk in terms of dollars or rocks. They'll say "$100 (£70) every 24 hours" or "six rocks a day". That's a drug culture term used by someone who didn't do the preparation himself.

'Crack has become very much a contributor to sexually transmitted diseases because of the prostitutes, the so-called "crack whores". They use crack cocaine repeatedly to the point that they are offering sex for a rock. They are in a cycle of drug use that, for many, is impossible to break.'

Asking addicted crack users about their habit is, to say the least, difficult. The drug makes them secretive, suspicious and hostile. Unless you're offering them more crack (and I wasn't) they don't want to know. But one Miami, Florida, user four months into treatment at least agreed to explain the lure of the drug. He was in real estate, young, wealthy and a former powder coke user. A business acquaintance showed him how to heat crack on aluminium foil and inhale the fumes.

'If you haven't experienced crack you can't know what ultimate pleasure feels like,' he said. 'It goes beyond any other human experience; you can't even begin to compare it to an orgasm. The first couple of minutes are a new level of consciousness. Your senses are alive in a way you cannot understand.

'After this you get maybe 10 to 15 minutes of feel-good feeling. Then you start to come down and it's a heavy down. You feel depressed big-time, tired and anxious. You know that the quickest way to deal with it is to smoke more crack and so that's what you do. And gradually the highs don't seem quite so high but the lows just keep getting lower. I did this on and off for six months and I was spending God knows how many hundreds of dollars. But at the time I wouldn't have said I was addicted.'

Another recovering user, a successful 27-year-old American record producer, tells how, while smoking crack, he would sit by his phone ready to dial up the US emergency services. 'It got so bad and out of control that I would pick up the phone, dial 9-1 then fire up the pipe and if I felt like I was going to pass out I would hit the other 1,' he told the Utah newspaper the *Desert News* (25 March 2002).

This guy, identified only as Terry H, gave away his Jeep and 50 bucks (£35) to a homeless vagrant on the promise of some crack. Sometimes he would rent a car and wake up in it three days later, out of gas and no clue as to where he was. 'I probably just let it sit there and idle out and not know it,' he said. 'It was the perpetual lost weekend.'

Crack, like all addictive drugs, operates insidiously. Whether or not you believe the 'one-puff-and-you're-hooked' line peddled by some media companies, the truth is that if you smoke enough it will get you in the end. The trick is knowing when to stop, when to know you're on the verge of addiction. It's a trick few manage without help.

THE DOWNWARD SPIRAL

An article carrying the by-line Sarah Merchant in the London *Sunday Times* (3 March 2002) illustrates this well. Fresh from Bristol University, Merchant moved to London to start work as a television researcher. She soon found that both old and new friends – professional types such as lawyers, bankers and advertising executives – seemed fascinated by cocaine. Soon she was doing a few lines. Then after a year or so she was invited to a crack den, a seedy drinking club in Soho, where the 'charming' host shared a pipe of crack with her in a back room. She didn't know what it was, but found the experience 'absolutely fantastic'.

She tells how she smoked crack occasionally after that, managing to stay on top of her job and enduring only the odd murmur of concern from close friends. 'Then I nose-dived,' she wrote. 'I was going to the bar a lot, several times a week, and would head straight into the back room with the host who by this time was a gibbering, jittering idiot. I remember one night seeing him on his hands and knees, looking for the nonexistent remnants of the crack he was convinced he had spilt. He was

> Cocaine causes repeated microscopic strokes in the brain leading to dead spots in the brain's nerve circuitry. *Treating The Brain In Drug Abuse*, National Institute on Drug Abuse, September 2000

desperate and paranoid. While I sat there waiting for a hit I saw a rat scurrying along a shelf above his head.'

She goes on to describe her descent into addiction, lone visits to the Soho club, driving to other crack houses at fashionable west London addresses, scoring the drug day after day. After a week of this, she tells of waking up on a beautiful day in her flat feeling 'as disconnected and empty as it is possible to be', no emotion, no purpose, a sense of insignificance. Frightened and confused she packed her bag and went back to her parents.

'It wasn't until I got home that I realised what had happened – I had become a crack addict,' she wrote. 'The thought was terrifying: I had always thought that I had been in control. How had I been so stupid? I guess I'd thought that since I hadn't felt "addicted" after the first hit, as we'd been warned we would, that I was never going to be. A big error of judgement.'

Yet despite this horrific story she concludes by admitting that she continues to smoke crack as 'an occasional treat ... maybe twice a year'. She indulges with extreme caution, she says, and knows now that she is in control. Any drug therapist reading her words will have smiled a sad smile. Crack versus human will-power is a terrible mismatch.

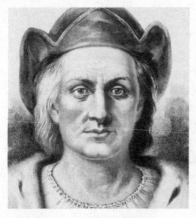

Italian explorer Christopher Columbus (1451–1506). Explorers in the Americas kept detailed diaries which reveal fascinating early impressions of coca. During his fourth voyage, in 1502, Columbus recorded how one of his lieutenants, returning from a river trip inland, had encountered a tribe leader with 20 men, all of whom never ceased chewing a dry herb and taking a sort of powder, 'which singular custom astonished our people very much'.

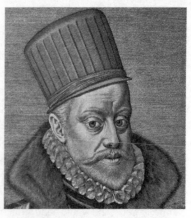

Portrait of King Philip II of Spain (1527–98). While coca was a poor export product from Spanish colonies (it rotted too easily), the Spanish cultivated it to sustain the labour of their Indian workers in the Bolivian silver mines. In 1548, the miners of Potosí chewed their way through more than 1kg million (almost 1,000 tons) of coca. Plantations pushed up production to meet demand and the Spanish mine owners grew rich.

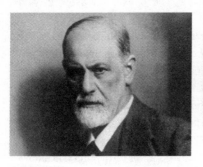

Austrian psychoanalyst Sigmund Freud (1856–1939). In 1884, Freud wrote to his fiancée, Martha, 'I have been reading about cocaine, the essential constituent of coca leaves, which some Indian tribes chew to enable them to resist privations and hardships. A German has been employing it with soldiers and has in fact reported that it increases their energy and capacity to endure. I am procuring some myself and will try it with cases of heart disease and also of nervous exhaustion.' The paper he produced later, 'About Coca', described in less than scientific language 'the most gorgeous excitement' of cocaine. For 12 years, up until 1896, Freud was a regular user, and abuser, of cocaine.

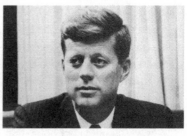

US President John F Kennedy (1917–63). In 1949, following a UN report, Cocaine production went underground, to Cuba – ideal for supplying the huge American market, run by mobsters Meyer Lansky and Benjamin 'Bugsy' Siegel. When Fidel Castro seized power in 1959, he deported the mobsters and soon disgruntled anti-communist rebels – wealthy from cocaine – were heading for Florida at the rate of 1,700 per week. The CIA trained and equipped these men as Brigade 2506, and on 17 April 1961 1,300 troops landed in the Bay of Pigs, southern Cuba, intending to fight their way to Havana. Within two days, the Cuban Army had killed 90 and imprisoned the rest. Kennedy was criticized by Republicans for failing to support the operation and by Democrats for allowing it to happen.

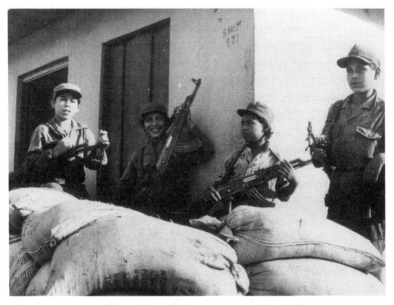

Sandinista militia in the town of Jalapa, Nicaragua. Behind America's interference in the Nicaraguan Civil War lurks the curious story of how the CIA turned a blind eye to cocaine trafficking – even using suspected traffickers – in its doomed attempt to deliver the right result in Nicaragua for President Ronald Reagan.

COCAINE IN YOUR BLOOD

My editor is going to hate this next bit. In the stream of e-mail briefings from him words like 'balance' and 'perspective' pop up all the time. The tricky thing when you're writing about cocaine and health is that loads of things appear on the 'bad news' list. So far I've found only one thing that makes you feel really, really good about this drug. And guess what? That's the feeling you get from cocaine.

Denying yourself something because it's not good for you may impress your mother but as a philosophy for life it sucks. Chips aren't good for me but I still eat them. Football isn't good for me (judging by the state of my knees) but I still play. Writing books isn't good for me because it hits my exercise regime. In each of these cases I make a judgement call and adapt accordingly. Maybe.

Unfortunately, cocaine is different, precisely because it's addictive. You might check out all the side-effects and decide it's worth trying. But if you become a regular user can you take a dispassionate view about whether to stop? You could ask enthusiastic cocaine takers what they think, although an opinion from the 'Drug Users are the Scourge of the Earth Society' would probably be just as valid. Asking recovered or recovering users might be more realistic, although, again, their perspective would be skewed.

The following examples illustrate the problem. The first comes from a special report on drugs, published in the London-based *Observer* (9 January 2000).

'Users and dealers, not surprisingly, claim it is less harmful than alcohol. Graham, a 34 year old whose Sussex seafront flat was bought with his earnings from cocaine dealing told the *Observer*: "Everybody wants coke. I think that's because people have realised that it doesn't do you any harm, not like ecstasy."'

Graham would therefore be surprised to read the following on the website of Cocaine Anonymous World Services (a self-help charity based in the USA).

'We went to any lengths to get away from being ourselves. The lines got fatter; the grams went faster; the week's stash was all used up today.

We found ourselves scraping envelopes and baggies with razor blades, scratching the last flakes from the corners of brown bottles, snorting or smoking any white speck from the floor when we ran out. We, who prided ourselves on our fine-tuned state of mind! Nothing mattered more to us than the straw, the pipe, the needle. Even if it made us feel miserable we had to have it.'

There is no way of knowing whether your cocaine career will mirror that of Graham and his mates or the Cocaine Anonymous addict. But, among health professionals and scientists, you won't find many arguing against the following statements.

1   Recreational cocaine use is never safe.
2   Some use it quite happily without serious health consequences.
3   Some use it and the health consequences are dire.
4   Some use it and die young.

A GUIDE TO THE SIDE-EFFECTS
The side-effects of cocaine fall into short- and long-term categories. Each of these can be subdivided into psychological and physiological effects. Sources for the information outlined below include America's National Institute on Drug Abuse (NIDA) website and Dr Mark Gold MD, distinguished professor at the University of Florida Brain Institute and a leading authority on addiction medicine (from both personal interview and published papers). While this section isn't really intended as a 'Spotters Guide to Coke-heads', concerned friends and parents of users may find it helpful.

POSSIBLE SHORT-TERM PHYSICAL AND PHYSIOLOGICAL EFFECTS
- A tendency to become talkative and energetic
- An apparent heightening of the senses, particularly sight, sound and touch
- A decreased need for food, water or sleep
- Dilated pupils, constricted blood vessels (the anaesthetic effect) increased temperature, blood pressure and heart rate
- Nausea, headaches and sweating

- Chest pain and breathing difficulties
- Urinary and bowel delay
- Large amounts (eg several hundred milligrams) can trigger onset of tremors, vertigo, muscle twitching
- Large amounts – regardless of whether snorted, smoked or injected – can lead to acute overdose effects such as heart seizures and strokes

POSSIBLE LONG-TERM PHYSICAL AND PHYSIOLOGICAL EFFECTS

- Damage to the nasal septum, causing nosebleeds, sense of smell loss and the 'cocaine sniff'
- Total destruction of the septum (single-nostril syndrome)
- Irregular heartbeat – leading to heart attack (rare); caused by increased oxygen demand on the heart (stimulant effect) and decreased oxygen flow to the heart (blood vessel constriction)
- Temporary paralysis of a limb
- Aortic dissection – the lining of the major vessel carrying blood from the heart tears under increased blood pressure
- Burst blood vessel in the brain (stroke) caused by increased blood pressure
- Overcompensation for the anaesthetizing effect on vocal chords, causing permanent hoarseness
- Bulging eyes; gaunt appearance
- Heart valve disease (linked to needle users)
- 'Black lung' and severe phlegm (crack smoking)
- Increased risk of HIV/hepatitis C (see below)

POSSIBLE SHORT-TERM PSYCHOLOGICAL EFFECTS

- Intense euphoria, sense of well-being, total control over destiny – the 'Superman Syndrome'
- Increased libido (low doses)
- Decreased problem-solving ability
- Restlessness, irritability, vertigo and suspicion of others
- A sense of doom and being out of control (during the crash); feelings of anxiety and panic

■ Obsessive behaviour – eg crack smokers picking at scabs or hunting for cocaine fragments

POSSIBLE LONG-TERM PSYCHOLOGICAL EFFECTS
■ Coke 'bugs' – a form of cocaine toxosis in which the sufferer believes insects or snakes are crawling beneath his/her skin
■ Hallucinations
■ Dulling of emotions and feelings of 'natural' pleasure
■ Intense paranoia; a mistrust even of family and friends
■ Feelings of isolation
■ Suicidal thinking and behaviour
■ Feelings of impending death
■ An (unproven) link to Parkinson's disease

SNIFFING OUT THE STATISTICS
In looking over this list it seems incredible that the 'cocaine is safe' lobby ever gets taken seriously. Measured in the numbers of deaths, you could perhaps argue that the drug has a low mortality risk (which is not the same thing at all), but official drug-related death statistics don't paint the full picture.

In America, hospital emergency room deaths linked to cocaine are running at around 10 per 1,000, a figure that has remained fairly constant for a decade. In Britain, however, the number of cocaine-related deaths has risen alarmingly from 19 in 1995 to 87 in 1999. Is this because there were more users? Are post-mortem detection techniques better? Are coroners being more forthright in their conclusions? At the University of Florida's Brain Institute, Dr Mark Gold believes cocaine death rates are a poor indicator of the true problem.

'When you look at coroners' reports they often don't tell you precisely what the person died of,' he said. 'Maybe they want to protect the family, sometimes they don't have the right tests to make a diagnosis absolutely and other times they just don't bother reporting the detail at all.

'I'm sure there are people around who'll say that powder cocaine isn't really a problem. It would be very hard to find a professor in any faculty in the United States who agrees with that. If you look at the people who smoke and inject cocaine, they started by doing something. We've seen people here who have become addicted to drinking cocaine as a means of weight loss.

'That doesn't mean everyone becomes addicted. None the less, the problems associated with this drug are very great. We've all heard stories of grandmothers who smoked for 80 years and never got lung cancer so it doesn't surprise me that people come up with single-case studies to show that cocaine is really OK.

'Here we have a drug which can hijack the brain, which in essence creates itself as the new drive state. Most experts would say that, particularly when smoked, its specific interaction with the reward circuitry is both unique and compelling. This is why when they take it people feel great, powerful, omnipotent – like the typical laws of nature don't apply to them. If you accept the original dopamine hypothesis you'd say that in the cascade of brain rewards cocaine comes closest to the endgame. It's the ultimate reward.'

Studies of 'crack babies' from similar social backgrounds show that exposure to cocaine in the womb reduces IQ by an average of 3.3 points. Researchers at Brown University, Providence, Rhode Island, estimate that the number of US children who later need special classroom help as a result of their exposure is 80,550 per year, at a cost of up to $352 million (£240 million) per year.

He points out that the long-term effects of the drug are poorly understood. Heart problems, heart attacks and strokes are all under suspicion, but suspicion and proof occupy different medical galaxies. Even tobacco has only relatively recently been branded harmful by the Surgeon General – 300 years after it arrived in Europe. Gold says that the most common cause of strokes in young people used to be tumours and 'arterial venous malformations'. Now, according to new British research, the commonest causes are cocaine, amphetamines and ecstasy.

'We need more long-term research,' he said. 'Medicines are viewed by everyone as dangerous until proven absolutely and completely safe and effective. And so we let the pharmaceutical companies and governmental agencies do extensive tests. Everyone complains about how long this takes but you do need 10 or 20 years to bring a drug to market.

'Then you have the drugs of abuse, which are viewed by many as safe until proven dangerous. With cocaine there's no silver bullet to treat addiction. Some groups are looking at vaccines and we've been trying a pharmacological approach without great success. We've also treated addicts who are health professionals – doctors, nurses and the like – and in that setting we use group therapy and support. But if you compare the doctor who's an alcoholic with the doctor who's a cocaine addict, the outcome for the cocaine addict is worse.'

LOOKING FOR A CURE
The quest for a cocaine cure has made some progress. NIDA researchers have focused on dopamine, seratonin and another neurotransmitter – norepinephrine – to produce genetic clones of their various transporters. The hope is that drugs can be designed to chemically alter transporters so that they resist the attachment of cocaine molecules. This would prevent the euphoria of a coke rush. Another idea is to disrupt the mechanisms of cocaine and neutralize it in the blood before it even reaches the brain.

Alternative therapy is also making a case. A study of auricular acupuncture at Yale University, published in the *Archives of Internal Medicine* journal (August 2000), involved the insertion of needles into the outer ears of 82 volunteer addicts. The group was treated for 45 minutes five times a week and, after two months, was tested for cocaine use. More than half the patients returned negative urine samples compared to 23 per cent and 9.1 per cent in two control groups.

Until a major breakthrough comes, most recovering addicts will have to make do with antidepressants and one-step-at-a-time group therapy similar to the process endured by alcoholics. The essence is to concentrate on avoiding cocaine for a day at a time – even ten minutes at a time – and to reject thoughts of tomorrow. Isolation from cocaine-taking friends and old haunts is key to the strategy because any reminder of coke can trigger its craving.

COKE-AHOLICS ANONYMOUS

This is where the other war on drugs is being fought – a quiet, low-key war in which staying clean 'just for today' is a major victory. At the Haight-Ashbury Free Clinic, Dr David Smith can relate directly to his patients because he himself survived an alcohol problem during the mid-1960s. He hasn't had a drink since, though he still occasionally attends Alcoholics Anonymous meetings.

'We have what's called the 12-step recovery programme,' he said. 'This starts with us asking addicts to admit they are powerless over the drug. That's the first step. Black users often tell us that they take cocaine because it gives them power. We say look, we're not saying you're powerless over your life. You're powerless over the drug. It's an important distinction.

'What happens with addiction is that first you get hooked spiritually, then psychologically and then physically, and so your recovery has to work in reverse. Once we have dealt with the physical and psychological parts we need to get the patient into a peer group in which drugs are not the medium of exchange. With black culture in the US, for example, there is a strong association with the Church so we work with churches. Our counsellors will maybe ask black users what they think about genocide – wiping out their own culture by dealing in crack. This is something that registers with them. It's one more reason to fight back.'

Dr Bill Jacobs is another specialist in the front line, offering courts the option of therapy for defendants as an alternative to prison. As medical director of two leading not-for-profit drugs agencies (Gateway Community Services in Jacksonville, Florida, and the Stewart Marchman Centre, Daytona Beach) he oversees treatment for between 2,000 and 3,000 people on any given day. Around half have used cocaine.

'I see a progression in the disruption of a cocaine addict's life,' he said. 'Usually the job is the last thing to go. First they suffer spiritually and emotionally. Then the family becomes affected. Then their close friends, interests and hobbies all disappear. But they tend to hang on to the job and I think part of that is a way of justifying that they're OK. As long as they're able to get up in the morning and go to work then they don't perceive a problem. That is the way addiction disease works.

'In this country we've seen a move from powder cocaine, which is a white, upper-middle-class drug, towards crack, an inner-city, urban African-American phenomenon. These days it cuts across all racial and socio-economic lines. It is now a fairly regular occurrence that in my residential treatment programme I will have a 65-year-old white female who is a crack cocaine addict.

'We are definitely seeing an expansion in the older population. It used to be that when we had someone aged 60 in treatment they were an alcoholic. They didn't use other drugs. Now it's wide open. Cocaine has an older, adult clientele. It may not be the first drug of choice but poly-substance abuse has become the rule rather than the exception.

'In the adolescent population the incidence has, in the last three to four years, declined with the rise of MDMA [ecstasy]. Crack cocaine has become more of an in-stage drug, by which I mean that adolescents have a longer drug history before they get to it. Once they are in their mid-twenties it doesn't seem to be quite so dramatic that they have to go through everything before they get to crack.

'I believe this is a perceived risk phenomenon. Every time perceived risk for a particular drug goes up, you'll see use diminish in the adolescent population. This works vice versa. Crack cocaine still has a stigma associated with it because it is just so addictive. When you hit a crack pipe you are administering a needle-less injection directly into the brain, which takes effect inside ten seconds. Any fast onset to the reward pathways of the brain encourages a higher addictive potential.'

The notion of perceived risk is worrying. Crack cocaine may carry a stigma but if it's the norm within a peer group this won't be a barrier. According to Aidan Gray at COCA many users are unaware of even basic health issues – let alone the different addictive characteristics of crack and powder coke.

THE UNPALATABLE FACTS
'When you're taking a drug you never want to understand the full consequences and dangers involved,' he said. 'It's pissing on the bonfire, it spoils the high. There's this strong image that powder coke is OK, it's pure, it's fine, but there's also this thing about the word "cocaine". I've

come across people saying, "I just take cocaine. I don't do crack." Very often they are playing with words.

'Ask people how they're taking cocaine and some will say they snort it. Others will say they smoke it in a spliff [cigarette]. Once you understand the

> Between 75 per cent and 85 per cent of regular cocaine users will suffer a psychiatric disorder at some time in their lives. 'Clinical Aspects Of Cocaine And Crack', Gold and Herkov

chemistry of powder cocaine you realise its vaporization level is high. It's not effective to smoke it – in fact it's a waste. What these people are actually smoking is either freebase or, more likely, crack. It becomes clear when you hear them describe the process they use: "I get the crystal out, I crush it down I sprinkle it in the spliff." This is all about terminology. Users speak the language of their peers.

'There are a number of dance clubs where people openly do crack and freebase. Everyone calls it cocaine and technically, of course, they're right – it is. That's the term they've learnt. But this group is not getting any attention from drug agencies and neither are they getting independent information. I've worked exclusively with cocaine users longer than most professionals in this country – since 1994 – and what I've come across is incredible ignorance. There's been a load of initiatives in the UK on the dangers of heroin, safer use, all that kind of stuff. But there's been nothing like that for crack and cocaine.'

Gray's comments have massive implications for cocaine users everywhere. Over the years part of the drug's appeal has been that it is quick, clean and simple to take. In contrast, the AIDS epidemic has reinforced perceptions that needles represent a seedy, dangerous lifestyle. If you smoke or snort coke there can't be an infection problem with HIV or hepatitis C, right? Wrong.

'When you snort cocaine it damages the mucus membranes inside your nose, where the drug is being absorbed into the bloodstream,' said Gray. 'The more snorting you do, the more you damage the septum. When that damage is done your nose bleeds frequently. It's a classic sign of a cocaine user that they will blow their nose and produce fresh blood.

'Imagine you're at a party. There's a group of people ready to take cocaine and they're telling themselves: "This is a safe drug, it's not in the same league as, say, heroin." So there'll be someone drawing up the lines and that person will often be the first to take a snort. If he or she is a regular snorter you could have fresh blood at the end of the straw. It's commonplace for the straw to be passed on – especially if it's in the form of a rolled-up banknote. There's some stupid thing about trust, about passing the note around the group.

'If there's another regular in the group then the chances are there'll be fresh blood to fresh blood contact. Hepatitis C, according to the latest tests from Australia, can stay alive outside the human body for up to three months. The risks are obvious. It's like sharing a needle, and of course injecting cocaine with somebody else's needle is another route for this disease to enter the body.

'The third route is smoking. People will quite often burn their fingers using a lighter. The type of crack pipe is important – some of them burn your lips or cut your mouth – and actually smoking crack cocaine dehydrates you a hell of a lot. One of the things you notice about someone emerging from a crack house is that their lips are really chapped. There's something about cocaine that makes people pick at broken skin or sores. They've got open weeping wounds on their mouths and they're passing around a crack pipe. Again, they can be passing on hepatitis C.

'Crack cocaine, because of the way it works on the brain, creates an incredible compulsion among users. You may know about the dangers but you ignore them. You get instances of people injecting cocaine and saying "I don't care if it's a dirty spike; I don't care if you've got HIV. I just want my hit." That attitude is increasing. We have to wait and see what the impact will be on HIV and hepatitis C statistics among cocaine users. The tragedy is that – especially among the snorters – there are a lot of people out there unaware of the risks.'

Coke and HIV is a nagging worry for public health workers. Not just because cocaine offers the disease a route into the body but because of the biochemistry that unravels once it's there. A study by scientists at the University of California Los Angeles (published by NIDA, 15 February 2002) looked at the direct relationship between drug and virus and discovered a 'double whammy' effect.

The researchers took mice genetically bred to have no immune system and injected them with human cells. They then infected the cells with HIV, gave half the animals daily liquid injections of cocaine and the other half a saline solution. Ten days later they found that the cocaine mice had a 200-fold increase in HIV-infected cells coupled with a nine-fold decrease in CD4 T-cells – the cells HIV attacks to destroy its host's immune system. In other words, cocaine helps HIV to breed as it destroys the body's natural defence against the virus. Given that crack smoking and prostitution often go together, the implications are obvious.

Gray believes that governments and drug agencies should be doing more to identify cocaine addicts at an earlier stage in their illness. 'Part of the problem is that addicts do not come into services until they're in crisis,' he said. 'You'll see heroin users because they'll at least come in to get clean needles, and you can help them stabilize and manage their dependency. With crack and cocaine you'll usually see people only when the shit has really hit the fan, they're on the doorstep saying, "I need help and I need it now." We haven't got a lure to get them into services. We give out needles but we don't give out crack pipes. Maybe we should.'

Keeping cocaine addicts clean of the drug is now a huge industry. But while the theory of recovery is similar worldwide, the style can be worlds apart. If you're rich, boy can you enjoy therapy in style. If you're poor and readjusting in some backstreet halfway house, then humility is the word.

REHAB ... AT A PRICE

One of the world's newest and most luxurious rehabilitation clinics is Promises Malibu in California's Santa Monica mountains. If you log on to its website you'll find it set in stunning gardens fringed with palm trees. There are idyllic sandy beaches, tennis courts, a swimming pool and stables (where you can, naturally, experience equine therapy), and the chance to take guided walks in the hills. Lunch is created by a gourmet chef and celebrity guests such as Charlie Sheen and Robert Downey Jr can relax in the knowledge that their needs are serviced through a one-to-one ratio of staff to clients. The bill? Around $29,000 (£20,000) per month.

Inevitably, questions are being asked in the media. Under the headline 'Is Rehab A Rip-Off?' (14 April 2002) *The Sunday Times' Style* magazine pointed out that five-star country retreats are not absolutely crucial to recovery. Especially at that price. It quoted Nick Heather, professor of alcohol and drug studies at Britain's University of Northumbria, who suggested that luxury surroundings might even be counter-productive.

'There is a mountain of evidence to show that you get equally good results from outpatient treatment for one-tenth of the cost,' said Heather. 'People abuse alcohol and drugs in a particular social environment. Getting them to sit around talking about problems and then throwing them back into their old world, full of temptations and opportunities to relapse, is not helpful.'

'Ritzy rehab supporters argue that the clinics carry huge staff overheads and compare favourably in price with, say, a private heart bypass operation. Robin Lefever, a former addict who runs the £12,000-per-month ($17,500) Promis Recovery Centre in Kent, England, told *The Sunday Times*: 'I make no apology for it. I believe that your surroundings have an impact on the quality of your recovery. I know what it's like to come out of detox and be sent to a really grim halfway house – it's incredibly hard. Being relaxed and having time and the right atmosphere to think in is incredibly important.'

Perhaps both sides are right. All addicts are not the same and if you're a Hollywood superstar you might feel reluctant to shuffle along to Joe Public's group therapy session if there's a chance that fellow addicts will phone the press faster than you can say celebrity coke-head. 'Private hospitals have their place,' says Aidan Gray, 'though personally I think there's an assumption from richer users that because they're paying £2,000 ($2,900) a week they're getting the best service, which isn't true. In a way it doesn't matter. A big element in recovery is belief and if paying money allows you to have more faith in the process then why not?'.

For some cocaine addicts, belief and faith will never be enough. They need something more, something that strikes through the agony of craving to reclaim the humanity that once existed. It might be anger, pride, fear or loathing. With Jodie Stevens, it was love.

JODIE'S STORY

Jodie* has done most street drugs in her time. Marijuana, amphetamines, heroin, cocaine – all of these shaped her teenage years. For a long time she told herself she was exploring higher planes of spirituality, although now she thinks she was handling unfinished business from childhood. Whichever, her path led to crack cocaine. It almost destroyed her.

We meet at her flat. It's tidy, comfortable and the walls are covered with paintings by her seven-year-old son. It doesn't look like a crack-head's den and she doesn't look like a crack stereotype. She's 35, red haired and despite a few worry lines hasn't lost her looks. Over coffee she starts with a euphemistic reference to the 'issues' that dominated her childhood. It turns out that these centre on an absent, alcoholic father, a chronically depressed mother, a brother addicted to heroin and a sister who dealt cocaine for a living. There are better starts in life.

Once this is aired she doesn't mention it again. She is anxious that I don't think she is blame-shifting and insists that she used drugs for all the usual reasons – experimentation, feeling part of a crowd and, mostly, having fun. There was free, personal choice right down the line, she assures me, until crack took over.

She was first offered powder cocaine as a 15-year-old schoolgirl living in an idyllic, remote and rather too quiet corner of the countryside. She'd tried marijuana but this sounded more daring. Her recollection is that the anticipation and preparation was as big a high as the coke rush itself and over the next few months she became an occasional party user.

Within a year, things had changed radically. It was 1983, the new romantics were in town and trendy London was scoring a white cloud of best Colombian cocaine. Jodie had moved in with her elder sister in the north of the city and was quickly enrolled in a coke distribution service centred on the house.

'My sister was selling it,' said Jodie. 'I took coke all the time because I thought that's what people did in London. I was playing games, I didn't take it seriously. My sister would take it while she was cutting lines to put in the little home-made envelopes – there was this big ego thing that if you could fold the envelopes right you were in the know. I tried

* Some personal details in this interview have been changed to protect Jodie's anonymity

everything that was going: alcohol, cigarettes, hash and speed but coke was the one that gave me the buzz, the confidence. When the crash finally came I'd be on edge, full of apprehension trying to get somewhere though I didn't know where.'

Soon she was going out with a dealer and trading drugs herself. She'd work in the outdoor street markets, keeping a coke supply handy to see her through the day. Every hour or so she'd rub it on her gums. 'I was getting through a gram a day, which I felt was manageable,' she recalls 'I didn't even think there might be a problem. Everybody I knew was snorting it and drinking vast amounts of alcohol as well. Health was just not a consideration.

'When it became excessive I'd find my brain wouldn't stop. I'd be whirring all the time unable to relax − edgy. I had a motorbike and I would go off and visit people but I never could stay for more than five minutes. I'd have a couple of lines, a spliff and be off to the next person. I could never stop still, never be anywhere. Certainly never alone with myself.'

For a time she worked as a motorcycle courier, later moving into the admin office. It soon became clear that her employers were enjoying a healthy tax-free income from coke dealing. The drug was available any time she wanted it and her boss's drawers were permanently groaning under the weight of cash. Despite this, Jodie doesn't remember thinking that powder coke was a problem.

In 1989 she moved to Amsterdam to live in a squat. Here she tried a pipe of crack cocaine, without knowing what it was. 'I don't remember feeling an amazingly intense high,' she said. 'Mind you, I was high on so many things at that time it was hard to know which substances were doing what.' Soon after this she met the future father of her two eldest children and they headed back to the UK to set up home. Having a baby at 23 was a watershed in her life and she resolved to steer clear of all drugs.

A study has shown that mean daily coca leaf consumption among highland Indians around Nunoa, Peru, is 58g (2oz). Men chew slightly more than women.

Her resolve lasted five years. Then she and her partner split up and crack came slowly creeping back. 'It became a problem because I wanted something to help me face the day − every day,' she said. 'Being straight didn't feel normal. I decided I really wanted to start using substances again and I felt it was better that the children went to live with their father.'

She dabbled in heroin and began drinking heavily. She also met the father of her youngest son and although he wasn't doing hard drugs at the time he eventually slipped into regular heroin use. Unable to feed or house himself he began living in a Salvation Army hostel in Bristol where he dealt and used crack cocaine. Jodie would go up to see him from her home in Devon. She says her aim was to hold the family together. But crack was available and she smoked it whenever she could. Over a few months the relationship fell apart and, on the advice of social services, she took her youngest son and moved into a women's refuge. Looking back, she recalls that time as 'total disconnection from life'.

'I knew by then that crack was dangerous,' she said. 'But it was like I was scrabbling to get somewhere in life and I knew I was never going to get there. So to avoid confronting the real problems I was doing crack all the time, as much as I could, each and every day as long as I could get money for it. I was binging and using heroin to manage the comedown and through all this mess I was still desperately trying to maintain links with the two older children. At one point I sat down and drew up a chart of past events hoping it would help me understand what was happening to us all.

'I would smoke crack and straight afterwards I would want some more. I mean, literally five minutes afterwards. I would beg, steal – anything to get the money I needed. Things that had once given me pleasure or emotional sustenance did nothing for me. I used to love simple things like walking in the countryside, you know, communing with nature, but I could no longer absorb any feeling from that. It's a slow torture. You end up with no friends, no relationship. You can't trust yourself and you can't trust anyone else. You come to see cocaine as your only friend. I think of it now as the deadening drug.

'When you're smoking it regularly, everything becomes uncomfortable. Even your body. That's why so many crack addicts don't wash – they don't like the feel of water on their skin. You can't maintain a temperature so you're constantly sweating hot and cold. There is only one way you can escape this physical discomfort and that means smoking more crack.

'At one stage I had all these awful lumps appearing over my tongue and at the back of my throat. I assumed it was because the rocks had been cut with something weird. But it didn't make me stop smoking. My need was greater than my fear. People I was with were really falling apart; they had open abscesses and channel wounds up and down their arms and legs. It reminded me of old horror films about zombies. Any human morals or scruples were completely cast aside. Crack addicts are like that, devoid of emotion. People talk about using cocaine as a question of personal choice but, eventually, choice is denied you.

'In my view it is more addictive than heroin, although heroin has more of a physical comedown. Every day I would wake up and ask myself what on earth I was doing. I could see that I was going to end up dead and yet every day I would carry on just as long as I could get some crack. I think what finally did it was the realisation that I couldn't love my children. Not didn't, but couldn't. It took months before I could feel any proper emotion. I remembered how love felt and I missed it terribly.

'For me it wasn't just the drugs. It was all wrapped up in my relationship [with her youngest child's father]. I felt I couldn't cope alone and I was fearful of being alone. The last time I went to see him he had a young girl who was a prostitute; she was there to get the money in. What horrified me was that the two of them together sounded like him and me. He'd say to her "Isn't it time you went out." He would put the pressure on for her to find a punter so that they could have more crack. I knew that if that was me I'd have lost all my children and I'd be there every day just doing a trick.

'I was smoking four or five rocks a day, whenever I could afford it. I was coming in and out of crack use, which meant I was generally taking less than those around me, and I wasn't prepared to sell myself to get money. I'd been down that road when I was younger and I knew I didn't want to go there again. This at least limited how much crack I could do.'

She resisted seeking help for fear that she would be classed as an unfit mother. She had visions of social services intervening to place her children in care; even denying her access. 'I knew what it felt like to be apart from them,' she says. 'If I'd lost that contact, there would have been no hope for me.'

Now her main goal is to 'get a good family life together'. She is doing voluntary work and trying to revive her love of painting. A local drugs project has sent her on courses to improve assertiveness and self-esteem, and this has allowed her to go shopping without fearing she would be accused of stealing. She is determined not to become a fanatical anti-drugs parent. 'If my kids told me they wanted to try crack, I'd give them my life story, tell them the facts as best I can and let them decide. The most important thing is to keep communications open.'

> Every \$1 (70p) invested in drug treatment saves \$7 (£4.80) in prison costs. Californian research, Dr David Smith, Haight-Ashbury Free Clinic

I ask whether she will be free of crack for good. There's a long pause while she considers this. She says she's been 'coming and going' from the drug for so long that it's a difficult promise. Even so, she's sure this time will be different. 'I've completely isolated myself from the scene,' she says 'I live on an estate where nobody knows about my past, my son goes to the local school and nobody I know is doing drugs. That's a complete turnaround from a year ago when I knew no one who wasn't doing drugs.

'It's difficult in the sense that if I looked hard enough I know I could find crack. But in this area I don't have the connections. There's no one walking in to the house and lighting up. People here don't know about my background and I want to keep it that way. *I* know ... and that's hard enough.

'I'm quite philosophical. I feel that part of my journey has been to plumb the depths, and part of me is fascinated by true deprivation and how low human beings can really go. I've been lucky enough to go down there survive it and come out again. Yes, I'm free of crack now because I can see it for what it is. I won't be controlled like that again.'

These are brave words, which suggest that crack cocaine really is in her past. Yet when I ask about the last time she smoked she admits it was ten weeks ago. Ten weeks! So the crack memory is still there, hunkered down in her mind, perhaps niggling away occasionally when she's down. It's hard to fight an enemy like that because it won't show itself properly. It relies on guile, and timing and ambush. Jodie's up for the battle at the moment because she loves her kids with unbelievable passion and they need her. You just wonder what will happen when they grow up and become more independent. Maybe by that time she will be truly free.

I hope things work out for Jodie.

> 'The United States asks peasant coca farmers to switch to fruit, which
> they must transport in vehicles they don't have, down roads that don't
> exist to sell in markets with no buyers. Even if there were customers
> the idea that the *campesinos* could compete in an international global
> economy is truly farcical. They wouldn't stand a chance.'
>
> – Sanho Tree, Institute of Policy Studies Drug Policy Project

THE MONEY LAUNDRY

Imagine you're a drugs baron, running cocaine from Colombia to wholesalers
and street dealers in north-east America. You've contracted-out the smuggling
and transport business to a Mexican cartel, which gets to keep a third of all
consignments as payment. You've bribed a few police chiefs and politicians
along the way and you've settled the pittance you pay coca growers. You're
share is still $1 million (£700,000) a day in profit. But there's a problem.

All your income is in cash – small denominations handed over by cocaine
users. The USA, along with most major western economies, insists that
banks report any cash deposit of more than $10,000 (£7,000) under a
process called Currency Transaction Reporting (CTR). Given that, according
to the US Customs Service website (March 2002), the total American
narcotics market is worth $57 billion (£39 billion) a year, and that there are
around 255 banking days per year, this would mean drug dealers depositing
around $223.5 million (£154.2 million) per day. Even if depositors managed
to make three drops a day without raising eyebrows there would need to
be 7,450 of them on the combined payroll. This is not the way drugs barons
like to do business. It would be a turkey shoot for the DEA.

Depositing drug profits like this sounds farcical but, actually, isn't. When the cocaine boom hit America – and specifically Florida – in the late 1970s, US Treasury officials discovered an anomaly in their sums. Why was the Miami Federal Reserve Bank reporting a cash surplus of $5.5 billion (£3.8 billion) in 1979 – more than the surplus of the other 12 Federal Reserve Banks put together? The answer wasn't long coming. All over the state, Colombian couriers were handing in dollar bills by the bagful. Some even turned up carrying cash in supermarket trolleys.

The Bank Secrecy Act (which enforced CTR) temporarily halted this practice. Then DEA agents began reporting a curious new phenomena in which dozens of cash couriers, each carrying amounts not dissimilar to $9,999 (£6,999), were being bussed around the banks on a daily basis. They looked so like caricatures – queuing to get off the bus, queuing to get in the banks, shoulder bags full to bursting – that the DEA nicknamed them after those much-loved cartoon characters the Smurfs. To this day, 'smurfing' is the DEA's technical term for multiple deposits of drug money.

There are dozens of methods used to launder cash but they all involve three essential steps:

1 getting the money into commercial financial systems, either through a bank or front company
2 'layering' that cash by moving it to different accounts (so obscuring the original source)
3 pumping it back into the economy as 'clean' money.

In theory the simplest way is simply to export drug dollars in bulk to a country where banks have no CTR. The problem here is that $1 million (£700,000) in small denominations is not easy to conceal. Customs officers deploy the same techniques they use to detect drug trafficking, even training sniffer dogs to recognize the smell of money. Latest DEA figures show a doubling of currency seizures (up to $12 million/£8.3 million at a time) from $38 million (£26 million) in 1995 to $77 million (£53 million) in 1998.

Given the risks associated with bulk shipments, some cartels set up legitimate businesses as cover. Flea markets and restaurants deal in bucketloads of cash and their legal earnings can easily be pumped up with cocaine money. Front or 'shell' companies (those that are registered but don't trade) are also popular, masquerading as art dealerships, precious metal brokers, real estate, hotel and restaurant businesses or construction companies. Fake charities and even religious organizations have been used as dirty money conduits and you could always buy a bank or corrupt its officials. But of all the methods employed by the cocaine cartels one stands out as a perennial favourite. It is the BMPE – the Black Market Peso Exchange.

According to the US Customs Service it works like this.

1   Colombian drugs bosses export their cocaine and sell it to wholesale dealers for US dollars;
2   They call in a Colombian-based money changer or 'peso broker', who agrees to exchange pesos he owns in Colombia for dollar bills owned by the cartel in America;
3   The cartel has now laundered its profits into 'clean' pesos and can get on with the business of trafficking cocaine;
4   The peso broker meanwhile uses American contacts to channel his drug dollars into the US banking system (some or all of the above methods will be used);
5   Colombian importers seeking to buy US goods and commodities place orders through the peso broker. He again uses his American associates to make the purchases, paying with the drug money now nestling in legitimate bank accounts;
6   Purchased goods – typically hi-fis and TVs, household appliances, alcohol and tobacco – are exported via Europe or the Caribbean, and then smuggled into Colombia, often through the Panama Canal free trade zone. The Colombian buyer avoids hefty state import tariffs and pays the broker in pesos. The broker, who has by now charged both cartel and importer for his services, then has more pesos to buy drug dollars.

So why is this a government problem? Black markets exist everywhere – not just Latin America – and still life goes on. The answer lies both in the

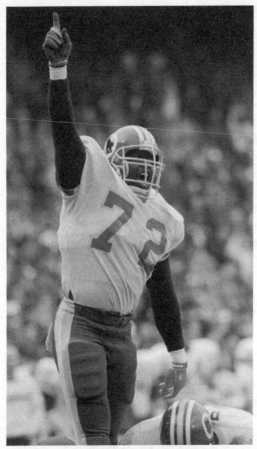

Drug testing has now become so prevalent in sport that for professional players and athletes a line or two of cocaine is no longer worth the risk. American footballer Dexter Manley (left and below with his wife Glenda in 1989) failed one test while starring for the Washington Redskins in 1989 and another two years later as a player for the Tampa Bay Buccaneers. He retired from football and eventually served 15 months of a four-year drugs sentence. In March 2002, he was again jailed by a court in Houston, Texas, after a drug bust at a city motel.

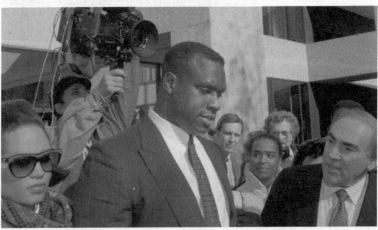

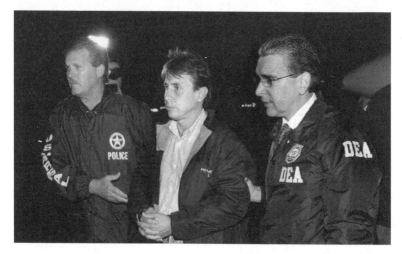

DEA agent and a US Marshal ushering alleged Colombian drug lord Fabio Ochoa upon his arrival in Miami, Florida, in September 2001. Ochoa, a former lieutenant of the late Colombian drug kingpin Pablo Escobar, was extradited from Colombia to face trial by a US court. Charges against him included participation in shipping some $5 billion (£3.3 billion) worth of cocaine into the United States.

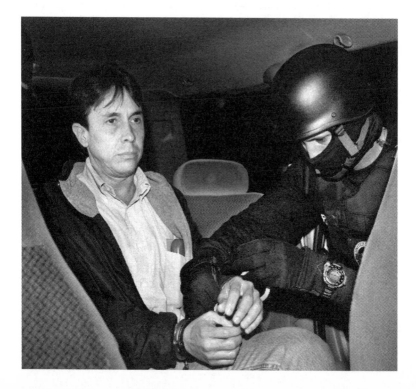

fragile state of developing economies, such as Mexico, Colombia, Peru and Bolivia, and in the astonishing amount of dirty currency swilling around the system. This is money that can't be taxed, buying goods that officially don't exist and paying wages that can't be traced. You don't need to be John Maynard Keynes to realise it's bad news for national treasuries.

INVISIBLE EARNINGS

Take Mexico for example. In 1997, before the recent government offensive against cocaine cartels, its drugs trade was worth $30 billion (£20 billion) a year – that's the equivalent of the rest of the country's gross national product (GNP) put together. The second biggest earner was the oil industry, which managed a mere $10 billion (£7 billion). By coincidence, $10 billion (£7 billion) was then the annual personal income of the drugs baron Amado Carillo Fuentes who, you'll recall, died undergoing plastic surgery in July that same year (London *Daily Telegraph*, 18 October 1997).

The Bolivian and US governments are pledged to eliminate all of Bolivia's illegal coca plantations by 2002, leaving 13,000 ha (32,000 acres) for domestic consumption (ie for use in traditional teas and medicines). Between 1996 and 1997, 63ha (155 acres) of Bolivian coca was replanted for every 100ha (250 acres) destroyed. International Narcotics Control Strategy Report

Among the $800 million (£550 million) per year handed out in bribes was the purchase of unfettered air access for Carrillo's drug planes. According to one contemporary legend he would take an hour-long 'window' in Mexico's air defence network and use it to fly through as many planes as he could – including a cocaine-laden Boeing 727. No wonder his nickname was Lord of the Skies.

Carrillo knew that his earnings were effectively keeping the Mexican economy afloat. He said as much in a letter to President Ernesto Zedillo dated 14 January 1997, which was later leaked to the press. 'Leave me alone to run my business,' it warned, 'otherwise I'll withdraw its benefits from the nation.'

US Customs officer Dean Boyd, who specializes in analyzing drug dollar laundering, believes Latin America is slowly accepting the need to challenge the economic muscle of the cartels. The BMPE, he says, acts like a parasite on a nation's wealth.

'This scam has been in place for decades; in fact it pre-dates the drug trade altogether,' he told me. It is just about the largest money-laundering system in the western hemisphere and primarily sucks in Colombia, Panama, Venezuela and the United States. The only way to tackle it is for these countries to act together using every agency at their disposal. Our best estimates suggest that BMPE alone launders between $3 and $6 billion (£2 and 4 billion) every year.

'Colombia is well aware of the problem and has been for a long time because it directly affects that country's economy. It results in a huge quantity of lost tax revenue for them because, in effect, goods are smuggled in as contraband and no import taxes are paid. This has had a devastating effect on their treasury and they have really stepped up their efforts to stop it. It isn't easy because a lot of the goods go through the Panamanian free trade zone. That can be hard to police. It is in the interest of the United States to help them because the end result is that our companies get paid in drug money. Nobody wants that.' There is certainly plenty of US help.

OPERATION WIRE CUTTER

In September 1999 the 'El Dorado' multi-agency task force in New York launched an ambitious strike against Colombian money brokers with Operation Wire Cutter. This saw undercover Customs officers posing as American-based money launderers to penetrate the Caracol cartel on Colombia's north coast. Over several months they picked up drug dollars in cities such as New York, Miami, Chicago, Los Angeles and San Juan, Puerto Rico, wiring the cash to accounts specified by the brokers. As the net grew bigger both the DEA and Colombia's equivalent, the Departamento Administrativo de Seguridad (DAS), were called in to monitor the dirty money emerging as 'clean' pesos and then as smuggled goods in Colombia.

On 15 January 2002, the DAS arrested eight brokers in Bogotá to face currency charges in New York. Between them they had 50 years' experience in the money-laundering business and allegedly offered their services on a contract basis to several different cartels. More than $8 million (£5.5

million) in cash and 400kg (880lbs) of cocaine was recovered. A further 29 people were held in various US cities (according to a USCS press release).

In a press statement released later, DEA Administrator ASA Hutchinson said: 'By integrating electronic surveillance with investigative intelligence, US and Colombian officials tracked millions of dollars laundered through the Black Market Peso Exchange and arrested the principle money launderers involved in the conspiracy.' Colombia's US ambassador was equally chipper, describing the operation as 'a model for how other nations around the world will have to work together if we are going to be successful in shutting down global narco-trafficking and terrorist networks.'

Wire Cutter was a major coup, although no one is pretending that it will deter the cartels for long. 'All we can do is make it as difficult as possible for them to use the BMPE system,' says Dean Boyd. 'What's amazing is that the traffickers are prepared to lose so much of their profits to these brokers. If I'm a cartel boss down in Colombia and I have $10 million (£7 million) sitting in New York I'll happily sell that for $8 million (£5.5 million) worth of pesos.

'That's indicative of how lucrative the whole business is. If we can make the cost of laundering more and more expensive then we are getting somewhere. Part of our job is to make life difficult for these people and if we can make them try another system then that's a victory. One thing is for sure. Whatever else they do, they always want to get their hands on the money.

'Typically, when we mount a major operation to disrupt money laundering they go back to bulk cash smuggling. That is a risky situation for them. Carrying millions of dollars in cash weighs a lot; it's very unwieldy, difficult to transport covertly and our sniffer dogs are trained to find it. After we complete an operation we alert our people on the borders to expect more cash smuggling and, sure enough, it always happens.'

In Europe the system works in exactly the same way, with drug money converted into various national currencies and cleansed through the purchase and smuggling of black market goods. Life may prove harder for the money launderers in future because the introduction (and inevitable adoption) of the Euro as a European-wide currency will make wire transfers more transparent. Until that time comes there's always Liechtenstein as a safe haven for dodgy money.

HAVEN IN THE HILLS

This little Alpine statelet has long been famous for its secretive banking, lax regulation and negligible tax regime. That's why crooks such as the disgraced (now deceased) British publisher Robert Maxwell liked doing business there. But in January 2000 a report by Germany's Federal Intelligence Service (FIS) painted an alarming picture of the extent to which the 160 sq km (62 sq mile) principality has courted mafia bosses and drug barons, including our old friend Pablo Escobar.

Ronald Reagan is credited with taking America into the longest war in its history – the war on drugs – in 1981. One of his first acts was to order the FBI on to the case, a strategy always resisted by its long-time director J Edgar Hoover for fear that drug money would breed corruption.

Through its 'cyber-spying' division, the Bundesnach- richtendienst (BND), the FIS claimed it had hard evidence that underworld figures across the world had been tapped up by men in suits from Liechtenstein.

It described meetings with the 'financial managers of South American drug clans' over many years and highlighted 'a network of relationships between high-ranking officials, judges, politicians, bank managers and investment advisers who assist each other with illegal financial transactions on behalf of international criminals.' The German news magazine *Der Spiegel* was rather more blunt: 'The secret document reads like the worst nightmare,' it fumed. 'An entire country in the middle of Europe appears to be in the service of criminals from all around the world. The findings destroy once and for all what was left of Liechtenstein's battered reputation.'

It should be said that in the wacky world of drug money, Liechtenstein doesn't have a monopoly on battered reputations. For all its talk of consensus and multinational approaches the White House has an undistinguished record of playing fast and loose. To test this statement you have only to consider the 'C' word. That is 'C' as in 'Contras'.

PLAYING POLITICS

The saga of America's cack-handed interference in the Nicaraguan civil war is well documented, unbelievably complex and mind-numbingly dull. Which is a shame because beneath it all lurks the curious story of how the

Central Intelligence Agency turned a blind eye to cocaine trafficking – even used suspected traffickers – in its doomed attempt to deliver the right result in Nicaragua for President Ronald Reagan.

A CONTRADICTORY CASE

The fiasco began in 1979 when the corrupt, family-run dictatorship of Anastasio Somoza was overthrown by left-wing Sandinista rebels. The Sandinista government immediately faced a new enemy in the form of anti-communist factions, collectively known as 'Contras'. Working on the basis that any group that hated commies had to be a good bet for America, the CIA offered $19 million (£13 million) worth of military support. Contra soldiers would be trained in Costa Rica and Honduras using 'Unilaterally Controlled Latino Assets' (ie foreign mercenaries). This meant the CIA could deny everything later.

There was just one snag. Congress was not in the habit of bankrolling the overthrow of legitimate foreign governments. Therefore the CIA had to tell a great big fib. It claimed that the $19 million (£13 million) was needed to stop arms being smuggled to El Salvador (another country developing worrying commie tendencies). When the truth came out in *Newsweek* in November 1982, Congress began the process of blocking Contra money. Two years later it emerged that CIA operatives had been busily blowing up ships in Nicaraguan harbours (including a Soviet tanker). This time Congress wasted no more time and the dollars dried up.

Reagan was furious. He still regarded the Contras as the 'moral equivalent of the Founding Fathers'. On the other hand senior CIA officers now regarded them as the actual equivalent of a leper colony. The agency skilfully shifted responsibility to the National Security Council, which appointed a senior marine officer, Colonel Oliver North, to take charge. He came up with the 'neat idea' of funding the Contras' war through covert sales of anti-tank missiles to Iran.

This scam went belly-up when Sandinista forces shot down a US C-123 cargo plane carrying guns and ammunition over Costa Rica in 1986. One of the crewmen was captured alive and the whole sorry story came tumbling out. Anyone who watched a TV news broadcast in the mid-1980s cannot fail to remember the 'Irangate' investigative hearings and Olly North's mantra: 'I have no recollection ...'.

Irangate should have marked the end of the affair. But then, on 18 August 1986, the California-based *San Jose Mercury News* ran a story headlined 'The Dark Alliance'. Reporter Gary Webb alleged that the Contras had funded their guerrilla activities by running cocaine to the USA, specifically Los Angeles, where it was turned into crack. Worse, that the CIA had known this and ignored it in pursuit of Reagan's aims in Nicaragua.

Over the next few years Webb's story was rubbished by government sources and rival newspapers. Most of them used the classic politicians' ruse of seizing on allegations Webb had never made and then 'proving' them inaccurate. However, John Kerry, a Democrat senator from Massachusetts, remained suspicious and in 1986 established a Senate Foreign Relations Subcommittee to probe further. Its conclusions, published in April 1989, were damning.

'There was substantial evidence of drug smuggling through war zones on the part of individual Contras, Contra suppliers, Contra pilots, mercenaries who worked with the Contras and Contra supporters throughout the region ... US officials in Central America failed to address this drug issue for fear of jeopardizing the war efforts against Nicaragua ... and senior US policymakers were not immune to the idea that drug money was a perfect solution to the Contras' funding problems.'

The Kerry Committee report went on: 'In the name of helping the Contras, we abandoned the responsibility our government has for protecting our citizens from all threats to their security and well being ... The credibility of governmental institutions has been jeopardized by the administration's decision to turn a blind eye to domestic and foreign corruption associated with the international narcotics trade.'

After much huffing and puffing the CIA eventually agreed to an internal investigation, which was so impartial it was carried out by ... the CIA. In December 1997 the *Los Angeles Times* acidly summed up a leak of the result as follows: 'CIA Clears Itself In Crack Investigation'. In fact this was not quite true. While the agency's Inspector General Frederick Hitz rejected the notion that the CIA actively trafficked cocaine, he found that it did allow trafficking to continue unfettered. In short, it didn't look too hard.

Paragraph 35 of the impenetrably phrased Hitz Report introduction reads: 'CIA knowledge of allegations or information indicating that organizations or individuals had been involved in drug trafficking did not deter their use by CIA. In other cases, CIA did not act to verify drug allegations or information even when it had an opportunity to do so.'

PANAMA SPAT

While 'Irangate' unfolded at home, the politics of cocaine were dogging the US in another particularly sensitive area of Latin America – Panama. This time the villain was one Manuel Noriega, a particularly loathsome bully who had been protected from child rape charges to rise to the top of the Panamanian armed forces. Panama had a reputation as a drug smuggling and money-laundering centre, but the Americans tolerated Noriega because he seemed to be on the right side. After all, Panama was acting as a pipeline for Contra guns ...

Estimates for coca production – and eradication – need to be treated with suspicion. According to the UN, 'cocaine output per hectare [acre] in Colombia is probably at least three times higher than reflected in US State Department estimates'. UNDCP, *Estimate Of The Value Of Global Cocaine Retail Sales, 1995–1998*, January 2000

Noriega was playing a dangerous game. He allowed Colombia's Medellín cartel to build a huge cocaine laboratory in the Darien jungle, accepting something between $2 and $5 million (1.4 and 3.5 million) in bribes. He also permitted the cartel to channel coke through Panama on payment of a $1,000 (£700) per kilogram (2¼lb) tax. Things started to go wrong when Panamanian army officers heard whispers about the Darien laboratory and staged a major raid to shut it down. The Medellín bosses are rumoured to have responded by sending Noriega a gift-wrapped coffin. The White House was more restrained but began to see clearly the monster it had helped to create.

As the 1980s rolled on, Noriega lost the plot completely. He had his main political opponent assassinated for publicizing the drug deals. He was accused by his second-in-command General Robert Diaz of stuffing ballot boxes to secure re-election. Stupidly, he began targeting US citizens in Panama as suspected illegal aliens. And, really stupidly, he hinted that American access to the Panama Canal might not be guaranteed.

By the time Panamanians began street protests demanding Noriega's removal, Washington was on the case. On Wednesday 20 December 1989, the US military launched Operation Just Cause against a man Senator Jesse Helms described as 'the biggest head of the biggest drug-trafficking operation in the western hemisphere'. More than 24,000 airborne US troops invaded Panama with the intention of bringing back Noriega to stand trial in Florida. Unfortunately, they couldn't find him straight away because he was busy in a brothel in Tocumen.

Soon after the invasion, Noriega tipped up at the offices of the Papal ambassador in Panama City demanding sanctuary courtesy of the Catholic Church. The building was surrounded by US Special Forces who spent a sleepless festive season blitzing the building with loud pop music. Noriega emerged on 3 January 1990 and was brought to Florida for trial. He was found guilty and will remain in jail for the foreseeable future.

You might think the lessons of Panama and Nicaragua would deter the White House from dabbling further in cocaine politics. You'd be wrong. The big three coca countries – Colombia, Peru and Bolivia – are all taking Uncle Sam's dollar as an incentive to restrict cocaine production. The hard statistics trotted out by the White House Office of National Drug Control Policy (ONDCP) seem encouraging.

LIES, DAMNED LIES AND ...
On 22 January 2001, ONDCP director Edward Jurith revealed that coca production had dropped 33 per cent in Bolivia and 12 per cent in Peru over the previous 12 months. Over five years the harvest was down even more dramatically – from 94,400ha (233,200 acres) to 34,200ha (84,500 acres) in Peru and from 48,100ha (118,800 acres) to 14,600ha (36,100 acres) in Bolivia. At a press conference, Jurith presented this as a major victory.

'Bolivia and Peru have demonstrated a sustained commitment to counter-drug efforts,' he said. 'Their ability to sharply reduce coca cultivation

159

illustrates that a long-term commitment and a solid strategy bring positive results. We look forward to continuing to work with their governments towards further reducing illicit coca production. These successes underscore that when political will is combined with comprehensive alternative economic development and the rule of law, drug cultivation and production will plummet. This is also our objective in Colombia where Plan Colombia envisions a 50 per cent reduction in coca cultivation in five years.'

Sounds like bad news for the cartels doesn't it? America taking the war on drugs to the enemy; being proactive instead of reactive; preventing a white wave of cocaine from breaking over its people. Doing something must surely be better than doing nothing, right? Let's probe Jurith's statement a little further. Let's start with 'Plan Colombia'...

This is a $1.3 billion (£0.9 million) military package introduced in 2000 by President Clinton to help the Colombian army destroy illegal coca plantations, fight cocaine trafficking and target rebel guerrillas in the country's heartlands. Over two years the Americans have provided more than 100 Black Hawk and Huey 2 helicopters, and hundreds of US troops acting as trainers and advisers. This intervention was a bold policy, which the European Union and most of South America refused to back.

> In 1990 Panamanian president and drug trafficker Manuel Noriega was trapped by US Special Forces after claiming sanctuary in the house of a Papal emissary. The building was blitzed for days with loud pop music, The Clash's classic 'I Fought The Law (And The Law Won)' ultimately clinching surrender.

European leaders were concerned that Colombia's appalling record on human rights had not been addressed. The 12 South American presidents (some of whom represented nations with equally grim records), meanwhile, reckoned that Plan Colombia missed the point altogether. At their August 2000 summit in Brasilia they argued that the USA should reduce market demand for cocaine, restrict the chemicals used in its production and do more to help peasant farmers grow different crops. Venezuela, Ecuador, Peru and Brazil all tightened security along their borders with Colombia, fearing a refugee crisis and a spill-over of military action.

In February 2001 the US Army delivered an interim report claiming that the coca destruction programme was going swimmingly. Nearly a quarter of Colombia's plantations had been destroyed in two months of aerial fumigation. However, commanders were cagey about the remaining three-quarters, most of which is jungle territory controlled by the powerful left-wing guerrilla group FARC (the Revolutionary Armed Forces of Colombia).

Since 1999, FARC has effectively governed a 3.8 million ha (9.4 million acres) 'de-militarized zone', offered by President Andres Pastrana in a desperate attempt to end the country's debilitating civil war. Known unofficially as Farclandia, the world's newest nation, it includes some of Latin America's most productive coca plantations. The problem for the USA is that FARC fills its war chest with drug money. It taxes paste makers and has set itself up as a monopoly buyer of coca leaf.

According to the *Sunday Telegraph* (3 September 2000), FARC earns around £600 million ($870 million) a year from cocaine. It controls 70 per cent of the coca fields and sets the price (around £700/$1000 per kilo/2¼lb of leaf). Although it has other methods of fundraising – Farclandia law 002 states that anyone worth more than $1 million (£700,000) must hand over 10 per cent for the rebel cause – it needs the drug trade for its political ambitions. It is unlikely that American crop eradication helicopters will be invited in to spray a genetically modified anti-coca fungus. As General Fernando Tapias, head of the Colombian armed forces, told the *Telegraph*: 'There will be peace. But first there will be war.'

FARC is not the only player in Colombia's coca market. Its sworn enemy, not counting the government, is the Self-Defence Forces of Colombia (AUC), which controls some 7,000 right-wing paramilitaries based around the bustling market town of Puerto Asis. This is also good coca country with around 60,000ha (148,000 acres) devoted to the leaf. Predictably, the AUC is equally cautious about its cash crop being zapped by US chemical sprayers. According to one peasant farmer in the region, Jose Sonza, 'the paras [AUC] are offering 2.4 million pesos [£800/$1,160] for a kilo of coca base whilst the guerrillas in the jungle [FARC] only pay 1.8 million [£600/$870]' (London *Daily Telegraph*, 24 August 2000).

The reality is that Plan Colombia may actually be fuelling coca production and cocaine prices elsewhere. On 17 February 2001, the British Broadcasting

Corporation (BBC) carried a report on its website that began, 'Fears are growing that Peru could soon regain its title of being the world's number one cocaine supplier. It is because of the huge US-financed anti-drugs operation in neighbouring Colombia.'

This report went on to reveal that new coca fields had been sighted in south-east Peru. It quoted the UN Drug Control Programme representative, Patricio Vandenberghe, who predicted that a shift in coca production from Colombia to its neighbours was a 'logical move'. A UN investigator, Humberto Chirrinos, said Peruvian farmers were being lured back to the industry as leaf prices rose 100 per cent – from \$2 (£1.40) to \$4 (£2.80) per kilogram (2¼lb) over the second half of 2000. This is basic economic stuff. Restrict supply of a desirable commodity and – everything else being equal – buyers will pay more.

AN UNWORKABLE SOLUTION

As the world's 'boilerhouse' economy, the United States knows all about wealth. What's not so clear is whether Jurith and the White House have got to grips with the politics of poverty. The idea that all South American coca farmers can switch seamlessly to new crops subsidized by US dollars is not credible.

Sanho Tree is a fellow of the Institute of Policy Studies (IPS), a respected Washington DC think-tank that prides itself on 'unconventional wisdom to public policy problems'. Tree heads the IPS's Drug Policy Project. He is scathing about White House claims of success in the coca fields.

'The eradication programme is absolute folly,' he told me. 'It doesn't take into account how much land there is for potential cultivation, nor does it appreciate the reserve army of the poor, the people who are prepared to defy the US and take a risk on growing coca.

'The bureaucrats are concerned only with Congressional mandates such as how many hectares have been eradicated in a year. They can't see that crop eradication is actually a great form of price subsidy. It takes a lot of coca off the market and ensures a high price for everything that's left. This is essentially what we're doing when we pay American farmers not to farm legal crops such as soya beans and maize.

'In countries like Bolivia, eradication has had a quite brutal effect on local people. This is because no money or thought is put into alternative development – or indeed any basic development. Bolivia is the poorest country in Latin America and it is now suffering great social upheaval.

'We have taken a relatively peaceful country and pushed it to the brink of civil war. Civil war isn't quite the right description because one side is well armed and the other has virtually nothing. But the *campesinos* [coca farmers] are now starting to ask, "Where can we get guns, we can't take this any more." They've tried peaceful protests, they've been shot at, they've been killed, and they are told to go and grow other crops that no one wants.

'The idea has been an utter failure. The United States asks peasant coca farmers to switch to fruit, which they must transport in vehicles they don't have, down roads that don't exist to sell in markets with no buyers. Even if there were customers the idea that the *campesinos* could compete in an international global economy is truly farcical. They wouldn't stand a chance.'

But peasant farmers are not all angels. They are allowed to grow coca for 'traditional use' and the White House is surely right to suspect that some of it reaches paste makers for conversion into cocaine. Again, Tree is unconvinced.

'Even if some legally grown coca is ending up in illegal markets – and I don't see much evidence yet for this – getting rid of it is not going to make any difference,' he said. 'Certainly not in terms of reducing street cocaine in the USA, which is ostensibly what eradication is supposed to be all about. Colombia's output is more than adequate to make up the difference and in Peru they're already replanting. The whole policy is a horrible failure.

'In Colombia FARC is now forcing farmers to grow coca whether they want to or not. Our interference there is actually helping to increase cultivation. FARC will fund their war no matter what it takes. They don't have a choice. I'm really not sure what the US government expects here.

'There is growing alarm in Congress about the transition from a counter-narcotics mission in Colombia to counter-insurgency and now to counter-terrorism. A lot of Congressmen are prepared to go along with the global war on terror because they're afraid to oppose it. But it is worrying that both parties, the Clinton administration, and even the Bush administration until recently, had promised the American people: "Don't worry, we're not getting sucked into this four-decade-old civil war. We're just fighting drugs." And now suddenly we're protecting an oil pipeline and we're fighting guerrillas and we're not looking at mission creep* any more, we're looking at mission gallop.'

Kathryn Ledebur agrees. As coordinator of the Andean Information Network in Cochabama she spends her time highlighting 'US folly' in Bolivia's coca fields. She says the American eradication programme –

'The CIA has now officially admitted that for 13 years it had a "memorandum of understanding" with the Justice Department allowing it, in effect, legal cover to employ drug traffickers and money launderers as agents, assets and contractors ... US government sponsorship of the Contras seriously aggravated the flow of cocaine into the United States.' *War On Drugs: Addicted To Failure*, IPS/LA Citizens Commission, May 1999

'Plan Dignity' – has been anything but dignified since it began in 1997. Instead there has been an escalating series of conflicts, culminating in the deaths of ten coca growers and four members of the security forces between September 2001 and February 2002. More than 350 other farmers have been injured or detained.

BITTER HARVEST

'The plan has targeted the very poorest people in Bolivia, the peasant farmers who grow coca leaf for survival,' said Ledebur. 'It doesn't significantly attack high-level drug traffickers or money launderers. The Bolivian government has eradicated huge amounts of coca in the Chapare [one of the main growing regions] but promises of alternative crops and employment are proving slow to deliver. As a result, levels of poverty and malnutrition in an already poor tropical region have soared.

'This is the first time the Bolivian military has ever taken a role in anti-drug operations. We have a country that has been democratic for less than 25 years and at a time when we should be strengthening that democracy

* Military term for the way in which politicians expand clear military objectives into a range of complex ones

we are instead creating strong, well-funded roles for the Bolivian military. There are conscripts who have to pull up the coca and there's a huge military police presence in the Chapare. This has led to a series of violent conflicts, many involving the so-called Expeditionary Task Force, which is a very strange group funded almost exclusively by the USA. These people are non-military; they are hired hands working under military command and they have been implicated in some of the most serious human rights violations to have occurred.

'It is true that nothing will be able to replace the income from coca in the Chapare but, as stipulated by the law, there needs to be something that provides an income for 35,000 families. What we've seen by aggressive US eradication is that they have pushed coca production around the Andean region. You have these big advances in Bolivia – it's heralded as the great anti-drug success – and yet Colombia is easily filling the gap in the market and Peru is planting again. We're actually seeing a net increase in the amount of coca grown and no noticeable impact on the price, purity and availability of cocaine on American streets.

'There is going to be a permanently funded US military presence in the Chapare. It will cost $10,000 (£6,900) a day to keep this force and that's roughly the cost of building a school. There is no exit strategy here. The farmers have no alternative so they replant coca leaf. Governments say that justifies a military presence. The coca gets pulled up by the military, the farmers replant and so the endless cycle goes on.'

These views are echoed by peasant farmers across the Chapare. One, Zenon Cruz, told the London *Guardian* (25 August 2000) how he had been forced to grow beans and oranges instead of coca. Plan Dignity meant that he and his family had to live on a fraction of their former income. 'My father sowed coca and his father sowed it before him,' he said. 'What the Americans do not understand is that this leaf is a gift from mother earth to our people, an ancient tradition. They do not understand its sacredness. They think it is all about drugs.'

More pragmatically, he added, 'You can fill a lorry with oranges and not sell any of them at market. But coca always sells like hot bread. I was making 150 bolivianos [about £20/$29] a week before they cut down the

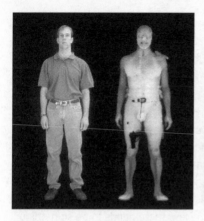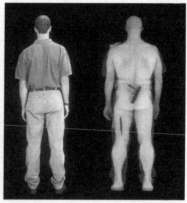

BodySearch X-ray surveillance displaying front and rear X-ray views of a male subject. Revealed on the front of the body are bags of cocaine (shoulder, waist); scalpel blades (chest); coin; metal gun; and plexiglass knife (LEGS). Rear view reveals bags of cocaine (shoulder, waist); scalpel blade and plastic gun (BACK); metal file and Plexiglass knife (LEGS). BodySearch scanning is one of the most advanced X-ray surveillance techniques, penetrating clothing to reveal soft objects – including plastic explosives – missed by normal security detectors.

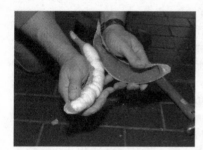

On 28 October 2001, police in the Belgium port of Antwerp found three-quarters of a tonne of cocaine packed inside fake bananas that had been included in a cargo of real fruit. A total of 756kg of the drug was uncovered in the haul found in a consignment sent from the port to Santa Marta in Colombia.

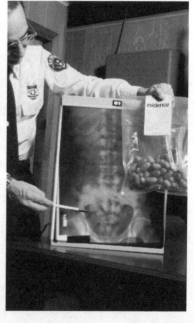

A customs agent in New York shows an X-ray of a drug smuggler's stomach and the recovered drugs.

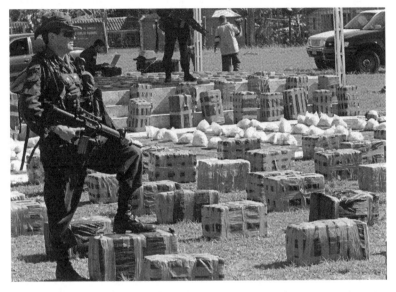

An anti-narcotics policeman stands guard in front of packages of cocaine that were confiscated during an operation in the port of Tumaco, in southwestern Colombia, April 2002. Three tons of cocaine, meant for shipment to the United States and Europe, were seized during the raid.

coca. Now we sometimes struggle to make 20 [£3/$4.50]. How can you feed a family on that?'

Another farmer, Celestino Quispe, was interviewed by BBC news in La Paz in June 2000. Reading his words you can't help but question the standard western government propaganda branding everything about the drugs business evil. Quispe patently isn't evil. Like most parents he's just trying to do his best for his kids.

'Coca is a means of survival for us,' he said. 'Because the soil is very tired, very eroded. Coca leaves are the only option we have for earning a living to feed ourselves and our families. We can't substitute it with other products like citrus fruits or coffee. Citrus fruits are very cheap. There are supplies sitting there rotting. I would not be able to feed my family by growing citrus fruits.

'Coffee is annual whereas I can harvest coca leaves three times a year. It does go down in price sometimes, but we always manage with coca. True, we have to replant every five or six years because the soil has to be renovated. But we can earn a living. You get much more money from coca leaves than you do for oranges. It's a very big difference in price. And oranges are heavy, so by the time you've paid for the transport to get them to the market there is nothing left for the producer.

'I have five children. Coca leaves allow me to pay for their education. My children are able to study, which I was not. I have little choice in what I can do for a living now but I am trying to make sure that they get qualifications. I would like for them to be able to choose what they want to do in the future. An education is very important because it will give them choice: they will be able to decide whether they want to grow coca like me or do something different, something better.

'Also, remember that coca leaves are not all bad. They are not only used to feed a habit. Coca leaves are also medicinal and a source of a traditional, legal beverage. There are no *cocalero* [coca grower] drug addicts. It is the gringos who have processed the coca leaves with chemical products as a drug.'

This is the argument now being drummed into a new generation of Indians. When families in Bolivia's fertile Yungas valleys gather to make their traditional offering to Pachamama, the earth goddess, they sprinkle coca leaves and alcohol on the ground next to burning incense. Their children then sing in Quechua:

Green coca you are born of our land
Your fragrance makes us sing happily
In the fields among the mountains
My little coca leaf is sweet medicine
Not a drug that does damage
We suck your juices for help in our work

For the poorest of rural Indian families, coca offers comfort in a harsh world. The irony is that their much-loved leaf – worth so much in the world's wealthiest nation – has never, and will never, rescue them from poverty. That's the sad thing about the cocaine business. The few who get rich are ruthless murdering bastards. Most of the rest stay poor.

BROKE ON COKE

Here's some food for thought. In 1969 the White House Office of National Drug Control Policy (ONDCP) spent $0.65 billion (£0.45 billion). By 1981, Ronald Reagan's first year as president, this had risen to $1 billion (£0.7 billion). In 1999, under Bill Clinton, it had reached $17.1 billion (£11.8 billion). This is serious money even by US Treasury standards. And still, every 30 seconds someone in America is arrested on drug charges.

One in five inmates in a prison is there for a drug offence. Almost two out of three Federal prisoners are serving time for drugs. The total annual cost of keeping drug violators locked up is around $8.6 billion (£6 billion). Counting the ONDCP budget (see above) that adds up to $25.7 billion (£17.7 billion) a year to 'control' drug use. God alone knows how much this increases if you factor in time spent by police, DEA, US Customs, the Coastguard, Army, Navy Air Force and assorted ranks of government bureaucrats. If you were running America would *you* call this drug control? Only if you were as high as a space cadet. (The above statistics were cited in Prof Craig Reinarman, *The Social Impact Of Drugs And The War On Drugs*, IPS, May 1999.)

Now relax. We are not about to plunge into the dreaded quicksand of social science. Besides, any argument that there's some neat and squeaky-clean answer to recreational drug use is absurd. No country has ever won a war on drugs, except accidentally when it happened to be fighting a proper war at the time (see Chapter 3). Even then success proved to be short-lived. As for decriminalization ... no, I can sense you glazing over.

> When the Mexican trafficker Alejandro Bernal-Madrigal was arrested in 1999 he told police he was capable of smuggling 30 tonnes/tons of cocaine through Mexico per month. *Cocaine: An Unauthorized Biography*, Streatfeild

However, cocaine's relationship with crime, poverty and – especially – racism in the USA is interesting. We know how scare stories of the early 20th century shaped hysterical legislation (remember the indestructible 'cocaine nigger'), but what's really scary is the way US courts still see poor, black, crack cocaine users as more deserving of harsh punishment than rich, white powder cokers. Scarier still is the view among many black community leaders that this strategy is right.

In the USA, sentences in crack cases are far longer than those for powder coke offences. Smuggling or dealing 100 g (3½oz) of powder attracts the same penalty as an offence involving just 1g of crack (cited, again, in Prof Craig Reinarman's report). Why so? It's the same drug. Crack is more popular in poor neighbourhoods (because it's cheap) but you can't start banging people up for longer just because their drug of choice happens to be popular. On that basis just about every American citizen would end up doing 12 years for marijuana offences. There is an argument that crack is more addictive, and more likely to provoke street crime, but then converting powder to crack is a cinch anyway.

Dr David Smith at Haight-Ashbury Free Clinic (HAFC) in San Francisco despairs of the 'lock 'em up' fraternity. 'I have found that politicians and public officials are often wrong but never in doubt,' he says. 'They will stand up and say: "You can't treat crack cocaine addiction. That's why we have to put them in jail." Well, actually, we have large numbers of successes with crack cocaine.

'Early intervention is the key. If you criminalize the drug, then this becomes so much harder. You can't tell some politicians that because they just want to lock up all the drug addicts. We are talking penny wise pound foolish here. If as a society we don't pay straight away we will surely pay later.

'We have a fundamentally racist system in that we put all the black crack addicts in jail and all the white cocaine addicts in treatment centres. There's been an increased government emphasis on criminalization and a decreased emphasis on early intervention programmes such as at HAFC. I actually don't include San Francisco in this because we're almost a different country as far as drug treatment goes. We have a much broader base of support for our efforts.

'Europe needs to learn from America's experience. We need to share this globally and understand the dynamics of drug culture. There is so much uninformed opinion that serves as a basis for policy. These epidemics and why they happen and what we can do about them – this all needs to be studied in an objective, professional manner.'

At COCA's UK headquarters, Aidan Gray is trying to do exactly that. He wants to influence political thought by igniting a debate on coke among politicians, police, health workers and anyone else who'll listen. Particularly users themselves.

'At the moment powder cocaine has almost a positive image in the UK,' he said. 'People who snort it are perceived to be rich and successful, whereas crack conjures up stereotypical images of users as poor, black, male, unemployed, violent people. If you look at the history of this drug you see very similar stereotypes appearing in American newspapers during the early years of the last century.

'At that time the US was prohibiting the sale of alcohol and opium to anybody who was Chinese, black, Hawaiian – basically anybody who

'Opiates and cocaine ... were first criminalized when the addict population began to shift from predominantly white, middle-aged women to young, working class, males, African-Americans in particular.' *Social Construction Of Drug Scares*, Professor Craig Reinarman, May 1999

wasn't white. So if you weren't white the only drug that was freely available was cocaine. It was handed out by the plantation owners and then the police said, "Oh these negroes are raping people left right and centre."

When you really study society and the history of racism you see the way stereotypes have been passed down and you begin to understand the sheer scale of the problem. But politicians always seem to skim the surface rather than tackle the underlying issue.'

He quoted from a US Department of Justice press statement dated 15 August 2001. It told the story of a Florida farm labour contractor called Michael Allen Lee, jailed for four years after using crack cocaine, threats and violence to enslave a gang of orange pickers. 'Lee recruited homeless African-American men for his operation and he created a company-store debt through short-term loans for rent, food, cigarettes, and cocaine,' the statement read. 'Lee then used that indebtedness, along with force and threats, to compel the workers to harvest fruit against their will. Lee admitted to abducting and beating one of his crew members to prevent him from leaving his crew. This is the fourth such prosecution brought in southern Florida in the last three years.'

Gray doesn't suggest that the UK's crack-poverty link approaches that of America. The racial divide is not in the same league, he says, although it undoubtedly exists. He pulls out a report from *Hansard* (the official record of House of Commons proceedings) covering a debate on London's Metropolitan Police (23 October 1992).

DIFFERENT RACE? DIFFERENT RULES

'Sometimes as a result of their own work, the police may gain a distorted view. For example, a recent Goldsmiths College report found that 79 per cent of known drug users in Lewisham were white, yet 50 per cent of those arrested by the police were black. Of crack users known to the police, 95 per cent are black, whereas 85 per cent of crack users known to other agencies are white.'

'Today the underlying issue in the UK is that cocaine isn't a problem unless you're poor,' Gray told me. 'You don't need to be black and poor. If you're living on one of the huge housing conurbations on the outskirts of, say, Sheffield or Glasgow, and you're taking crack cocaine, then you're a problem. If you're living in Notting Hill Gate [west London] and you're rich, then it's a bit of sympathy and off to the Priory [an exclusive rehabilitation centre] for a couple of weeks.

'In the USA, the Supreme Court has recently ruled that if you're in public housing in America and a member of your family is convicted of a drugs felony then the whole family can be removed from that house. You're a very poor family, your son or daughter gets caught smoking crack cocaine, you're trying to sort it out and suddenly you've lost your house. It must be a great help.

'This is about class as well as colour and ethnicity. It cuts across all drugs. But it's not exclusively about poor people and we sometimes forget that. If you look at the UK drugs agencies the majority focus on street use. Their opening hours are 9–5 Monday to Friday, which means that they assume users are unemployed. All the focus goes to unemployed users, the underclass. In actual fact the majority of those using cocaine in Britain are taking cocaine hydrochloride [powder] and they're working people or they're at college. Their needs are not addressed but they are surely just as important.'

In May 1999 the Institute for Policy Studies looked at the class-and-crack issue as part of its Citizens Commission on US Drug Policy, held in Los Angeles. These hearings brought together senior judges, law professors and prison reformers to take evidence from experts. One of the witnesses was Franklin Ferguson Jr, a black civil rights attorney.

'This problem begins not with race but with class,' he said. 'Like a range of other crimes past and present the drug trade consists of consensual transactions that take place within organized sales and distribution networks. These networks tend to segment by economic class. The rise of crack in the 1980s produced a class divide in the cocaine market that was unusually visible.'

He then listed the 'retributive' factors that have persuaded judges in cocaine cases to be tougher on poor crack smokers and dealers than they are on rich powder snorters and dealers.

'The former are certainly perceived to cause greater social harm than the latter and therefore seem to deserve harsher treatment,' he said. 'Lower-class criminal markets tend to be more violent than their upper class equivalents, at least in terms of the manner in which our society typically measures violence. It is easier to catch and punish sellers and buyers in lower-class markets than it is to catch and punish their higher end, white collar counterparts. The lower-class markets are eminently more visible. Lower-class constituents simply possess a much lower expectation of privacy, in direct proportion to their possession of land and property. This does not, however, justify the practice.

'Many have come to believe that because whites disproportionately use powder cocaine while blacks disproportionately use crack cocaine, a two-tier system of punishment has developed. The disparity between the amount of powder cocaine and crack cocaine required to warrant the same penalty for drug trafficking is 100-to-1.'

Ferguson quoted figures showing how the legal system's crusade against crack had significantly increased the proportion of black prisoners in US jails. In 1997 the prison population was estimated at 1,725,842 – 51 per cent of whom were African-Americans. Yet African-Americans made up just 13 per cent of the total US population.

Of the 2,100 federal prisoners doing time in jail for crack, 92 per cent were African-American, compared to just 27 per cent of the 5,800 federal prisoners sentenced for powder coke. Finally there's the 'killer' fact that sentences in crack cases 'average three to eight times longer than sentences for comparable powder offenders'.

> In 1982, 10.4 million Americans tried cocaine for the first time, more than in any subsequent or preceding year, according to a Drug Abuse Warning Network report. In 1998 there were 934,000 new users. US National Drug Control Strategy 2001 annual report

In his evidence Ferguson said: 'Even amongst staunch advocates of the black urban poor community there is support for this apparent disparity in enforcement. The crack trade destroys not only those who engage in it but also the neighbourhoods in which it takes place. Those neighbourhoods are filled with predominantly honourable black citizens who do not buy and sell crack. These citizens ... may benefit from sentencing and enforcement policies that target crack relative to other drugs since crack's residual, often violent, criminal activities are simultaneously targeted.'

In other words most black people living in areas rife with crack dealing don't care that the majority of arrests involve other blacks. Nor do they care about hefty sentences. They just want these people run out of town.

Naturally, politicians notice this mindset. Nobody, they tell themselves, ever got kicked out of office for talking tough on drugs. Locking up crack users is easier to sell to the voters than funding new treatment centres. Crack cocaine is good for scare stories and scare stories are good for talking tough. QED: Lock the bastards up.

SNOUTING OUT A SCAPEGOAT

This brand of political logic was addressed by Professor Craig Reinarman, professor of sociology at the University of California, Santa Cruz, at the 1999 LA Citizens' Commission hearings. There he delivered a paper entitled 'The Social Construction Of Drug Scares', which among other things considered that old election chestnut: the scapegoat. Scapegoating was defined by Reinarman as 'blaming a drug or its alleged effects on a group of its users for a variety of pre-existing social ills that are typically only indirectly associated with it'. Reading his paper you realise that, with some half-decent spin-doctoring, absolutely anything can be blamed on drugs.

'To listen to the Temperance crusaders,' said Reinarman, 'one might have believed that without alcohol use America would be a land of infinite economic progress with no poverty, crime, mental illness or even sex outside marriage. To listen to leaders of organized medicine and the government in the 1960s one might have surmised that without marijuana and LSD there would have been neither conflict between youth and their parents nor opposition to the Vietnam War. And to believe politicians and the media in the past six years is to believe that without the scourge of crack the inner cities and the so-called underclass would, if not disappear, at least be far less scarred by poverty, violence and crime.

'There is no historical evidence supporting any of this. In short, drugs are richly functional scapegoats. They provide elites with fig leaves to place over unsightly social ills that are endemic to the social system over which they preside. And they provide the public with a restricted aperture of attribution in which only a chemical bogeyman or the lone deviants who ingest it are seen as the cause of a cornucopia of complex problems.'

The truth is that crack cocaine is directly linked to poverty – both for those who grow it and those who take it. But it's not the *cause* of crime and poverty in the ghetto any more than powder cocaine is the *cause* of fraud and wealth on Wall Street. The distinguished Harvard law professor Derek Curtis Bok once famously observed that 'if you think education is expensive, try ignorance'. Ignorance breeds poverty. Ignorance of cocaine breeds addiction.

ADDITIONAL INFO

> 'Everywhere and at all times men and women have sought, and duly found, the means of taking a holiday from the reality of their generally dull and often acutely unpleasant experience.'
>
> – Aldous Huxley, *A Treatise On Drugs*, 1931

COCAINE: THE NEXT HIT

Cocaine will always be with us. It's better than sex (at least, that's what it tells your brain) and about as easy to ban. Given that it can't be uninvented, expunged from the face of the earth or chemically altered to be user-friendly, the only issue is how to manage its presence. The smart-arse answer is to try anything that hasn't already proved a failure. The overall result may not be a triumph, but it is hard to see how things will be worse.

In political circles buzz phrases like 'blue sky thinking' and 'thinking outside the box' are trendy at the moment Like all the best doctrinal clichés they have wonderfully flexible meanings. Even so, the clear impression delivered to voters is that shibboleths are OUT, creativity is IN and no idea is off limits. As politicians, police officers and editors raise the stakes in the war on drugs, we're seeing new initiatives taken up like nose candy at a Wall Street executive's leaving party.

Among the most radical of these ideas supported, worryingly, by both the liberal left and rabid right, is the decriminalization of 'hard' drugs. This book hasn't touched on this subject, because 'decriminalization' is an offensively bureaucratic word and the arguments for and against it are tediously polarized. Same applies to the debate on making drugs legally available over the counter. Let's get this over with quickly.

DOUBTS ABOUT DECRIMINALIZATION
The three big advantages cited in favour of legal use are:

1   the market for drug trafficking would collapse;
2   the police would be able to focus on other crimes;
3   users could be properly monitored and educated.

Sure, a few dealers would struggle on, undercutting state prices or offering something that bit stronger. But the real drug money would be gone for good. Coke use would be up front and manageable.

Unfortunately, from what we know about cocaine, there are moral and practical problems with these arguments. For a start, who's going to decide when a crack addict has had enough crack. Certainly not the addict – he or she will want to smoke until death intervenes. Of course, you may feel that crack-heads have a right to decide to die this way. But are they really deciding? As Jodie, the former crack user quoted in Chapter 4 puts it, 'People talk about using cocaine as a question of personal choice but, eventually, choice is denied you.'

Then there's the dilemma of younger users. Do we say coke is OK at the age of 18, 16, 14 or 12? What's wrong with a five year old trying it? Who decides on 'safe' purity levels? As soon as you dilute cocaine or make it off limits to anybody you instantly create a new black market. Maybe not so big, but still there. That means more trafficking and more policemen hunting traffickers. As for making powder coke legal but continuing to proscribe crack – please, do pay attention at the back there!

BACK IN THE REAL WORLD ...
Assuming that cocaine will always be with us and always be recreationally illegal, what might world governments usefully do? They could help America eradicate coca crops, making life harder for producers and traffickers. Harder, sometimes, but also more profitable (remember, destroying coca supports its market price). And not as hard as the life facing peasant farmers for whom coca is the only practical means of survival. Crop eradication as it stands is becoming more discredited by the day.

Perhaps the war on drugs could be intensified. More gunships and attack helicopters, more soldiers and armed agents, more nifty electronic surveillance, bigger rewards for informers ... all could inflict serious damage on the trafficker. But not all traffickers. And when you've hit so many that cocaine supplies become scarce, up goes the price and the profit, and in comes a new generation of millionaire coke kings.

There's the laughingly named deterrent factor, of course. This means locking up drug users and dealers for long stretches. It's great news for prison officers seeking job security but a real bummer for the rest of us who pay the bills. Drug users get to use more drugs in prison. Traffickers on the outside cheer loudly because the competition's out of action. As for the deterrent factor, there's not been much success there in half a century.

Finally there's that old favourite in the politician's armoury – the scare tactic. This essentially involves middle-aged, stressed-out people telling young carefree people that having fun is no good for them. All right, they can have fun reading or listening to music (quietly) but certainly not doing drugs. Alcohol doesn't count because lots of middle-aged, stressed-out people enjoy the odd drink.

Scare tactics never work in the long term. The classic response of parents to the first big wave of cocaine use that hit in the 1980s was to tell their children:

- 'You don't want to know about this';
- 'You will do yourself harm if you try it';
- '*We* will do you harm if you try it'.

Funnily enough, these responses pretty much reflected US government policy. Telling young people that cocaine will either kill them or get them jailed is not a sensible plank on which to base an entire policy.

Most studies suggest something like 80 per cent of powder coke users never report health problems. Users themselves aren't stupid. They know this. What they really need is clear, unbiased information about the true level of risk to the best of current knowledge. How much more effective would it be for governments and the mass media to put health risks into perspective. But then 'drugs', 'politics', 'media' and 'perspective' are not words that sit easily together in the same sentence.

As in most things, balance is the key. It's probably right to reduce coca crops as long as farmers are offered a realistic new living. It's right to lock up murderous traffickers and dealers, but sensible to keep addicts out of jail and in publicly funded treatment centres. It's right to stress the dangers of coke and also to accept that many users never become ill or addicted. If we are going to fight a drugs war let's at least stop truth becoming the first casualty.

Next time you're introduced to Charlie, by all means enjoy his company. But don't arrange to meet regularly. He can be *so* two-faced at times.

ABC OF STREET NAMES FOR COCAINE

(Note that this is not a definitive list; new street names are emerging all the time.)

Angie

Aunt Nora

Base (used for cocaine and crack)

Batman (also used for heroin)

Bazulco

Bernie's flakes

Big bloke

Big C

Bolivian marching powder

Bouncing powder

California cornflakes

Carrie

Cecil

Charlie

Cholly

Double bubble

Dream

Esnortiar (Spanish)

Everclear

Flake

Florida snow

Foo foo

Friskie powder

Gift-of-the-sun-god

Gin

Girl

Happy dust

Heaven

Her

Icing

Jejo

Jelly

King

Lady

Late night

Love affair

Mama coca

Monster

Movie star drug

Nose candy

Oyster stew

Paradise

Pearl

Pimp

Polvo blanco (Spanish)

Quill (also heroin; methamphetamine)

Ready rock (crack cocaine)

Roxanne

Scottie

She

Sleigh ride

Snow/snowbird

Speedball (cocaine/heroin mix)

Teenager

Teeth

Thing

Toot

Whizbang (cocaine/heroin mix)

Yeyo (Spanish)

Zip

GLOSSARY

Alkaloid – mind-altering nitrogen-based organic compound found in many drugs, including cocaine

Balling – vaginally implanted cocaine

Base crazies – people who search on their hands and knees for cocaine/crack

Based out – crack or freebase user unable to control usage

Beiging – chemicals that alter the appearance of cocaine to make it look as if it is of purer quality than it actually is

Bipping – snorting heroin and cocaine simultaneously

BMPE – Black Market Peso Exchange (method of laundering drug money)

Body packer – smuggler who swallows packets of cocaine

Break night – staying up all night on a cocaine binge

C joint – place where cocaine is sold

Campesinos – coca leaf farmers

Chalked up – under influence of cocaine

Chuspa – coca pouch carried by leaf chewers

CIA – America's Central Intelligence Agency

Cocaine hydrochloride – chemical name for powder coke; sometimes called cocaine salt

Cocalos – coca leaf plantations

Coke bar – pub or bar where cocaine is taken openly

Coke bugs – form of toxic psychosis in which cocaine addicts believe insects or snakes are crawling beneath their skin

Cooking up – processing powder coke into crack

Coqueros – coca chewers

Crash – feeling of dismay/depression that follows the cocaine 'high' or 'rush'

Cutting – process in which powder coke is chopped into lines using credit card or razor blade; process of diluting cocaine with other substances, eg glucose

DEA – America's Drug Enforcement Administration

Dopamine – chemical messenger in brain closely associated with euphoric feeling produced by cocaine

Drive-by shooting – popular gangland assassination technique in which the gunman opens fire from a moving car

Drug dollars – money earned through illicit drug sales

Flame cooking – smoking cocaine freebase by placing the pipe over a stove flame

Freebase – powder coke converted by chemical process to a smokeable form

Gak-blowing – taking cocaine anally

Ghostbusting – searching for any white particle in the conviction that it is crack

Hash – cannabis or marijuana

High – euphoric feeling produced by cocaine

Horning – inhaling cocaine

Iscupuru – container, often a gourd, containing llipta, an alkaline substance (see below)

Line – powder coke laid out ready for snorting

Llipta – alkaline, such as lime or powdered shell, used to leach out alkaloids from coca leaf during chewing

Los Pistoleros – assassination technique in which the gunman sits as pillion passenger on a motorbike; the favoured method of Colombian cartels

LSD – lysergic acid diethylamide – potent hallucinatory drug

Mule – smuggler who carries drugs in the body or in luggage

Neurotransmitter – chemical messenger that allows brain cells to communicate with each other

NIDA – National Institute on Drug Abuse (US research organization)

ONDCP – Office of National Drug Control Policy (based at the White House, USA)

Paste – crudely processed cocaine, often in brick form

Reinforcer – brain mechanism that urges that an action be repeated

Reward pathway – method by which the brain decides that an action is good and should be repeated; sex, food, warmth and child-rearing have strong reward pathways – none of these is as strong as a cocaine habit

Rock – piece of crack cocaine

Rock starring – sex with a man/woman who takes crack cocaine as payment

Rush – euphoric feeling produced by cocaine

Satiety – brain mechanism that decides when an enjoyable experience should end

Septum – area between nostrils, sometimes destroyed by prolonged cocaine use

Seratonin – chemical messenger in brain linked to euphoria caused by cocaine use

Shebanging – mixing cocaine with water and spraying it up the nose

Smurfing – laundering drug money by depositing large quantities of cash in banks

Spliff – cigarette containing crack cocaine

Stone – piece of crack cocaine

Synapses – spaces between brain nerve cells in which cocaine causes build-up of dopamine and consequent euphoria

Taxing – process in which one drug gang robs another

Yardies – general description for Jamaican underworld gangs

COCAINE: A LINE THROUGH TIME

Prehistory: Andean Indians discover properties of coca

12th century AD: Rise of the Inca; coca established as a key element of religious life in South America

1502: Columbus expedition makes contact with coca-chewing Indians

1532: Francisco Pizarro's private army invades Peru

1546: Spanish rediscover the silver mines of Potosí; paying miners in coca leaf becomes more widespread

1552: Roman Catholic Church makes first attempt to ban the 'evil' herb coca

1609: Contemporary accounts show that the Church is getting a slice of coca profits and no longer makes a fuss

1786: French biologist Jean Chevalier de Lamarck classifies the leaf as Erythroxylum coca

1859: Research student Albert Niemann extracts the cocaine alkaloid from coca, so 'inventing' cocaine

1863: Vin Mariani – a wine containing cocaine – is launched to wide acclaim in Europe

1884: Sigmund Freud begins experiments with the drug

1884: Freud's student colleague Carl Koller discovers cocaine's use as a local anaesthetic

1884: Freud tries to cure morphine addiction in his friend Ernst von Fleischl-Marxow by administering cocaine

1885: Fleischl-Marxow becomes the world's first coke addict

1885: American John Pemberton comes up with a cocaine drink syrup he calls Coca-Cola

1905: Amid mounting public concern, the Coca-Cola company removes cocaine from its drink

1914: The New York Times carries reports of a 'cocaine nigger' turned into a crazed killer by the drug

1921: The Fatty Arbuckle scandal highlights widespread cocaine use in Hollywood

1922: New laws in America impose ten-year jail sentence on convicted cocaine dealers

WWII years: Cocaine use all but disappears in America

1949: United Nations begins process of closing legal coke laboratories in Peru

1950s: Cuba emerges as the centre of global cocaine trafficking

Late 1960s: Colombia begins to challenge Cuba for control of world markets

1970: Rolling Stone magazine declares cocaine 'Drug of the Year'

1973: Pinochet gains power in Chile; hundreds of Chilean traffickers extradited to America

1975: Full-scale cocaine war breaks out between rival cartels in Colombia

Late 1970s: Pablo Escobar emerges as Colombia's most powerful drugs baron

1979: Huge cocaine money-laundering operation identified in Florida

1979: US officials begin covert support for Contra rebels in Nicaragua; turn blind eye as drug
running to America helps finance the war

Mid-1980s: Escobar's cocaine profits estimated at $1 million (£700,000) a day; number of
American coke users tops ten million; crack cocaine becomes widespread in USA

1984: Colombian anti-drug crusader and justice minister Lara Bonilla assassinated

1986: CIA-Contra scandal exposed by US press

1989: US launches Operation Just Cause against Panama's Manuel Noriega

1992: Escobar shot dead by Colombian police

2000: President Clinton launches Plan Colombia to wipe out coca plantations in the country

2001: Jamaica highlighted as new centre for cocaine trafficking

2002: British and European press highlight crack cocaine wars among underworld gangs

2002: Coca farmers battle US-backed forces eradicating coca crops in Bolivia

INDEX

acid (see *LSD*)
acupuncture 135
addiction to Coca-Cola 95
addiction to cocaine
  belief that cocaine is
    non-addictive 96, 104
  knowing when to stop 128
  long-term use and 53-4
  physiology of addiction
    118-23
  progression of 18, 136
  speed of delivery and 10
  'three Cs' of addiction 126
  treatment 37, 140-1, 170
Advertising Standards
  Authority (ASA) 19-20
AFO (Arellano-Felix
  Organization) 59-60
Africa 45, 48
Aherne, Caroline 28
AIDS and HIV 138, 139-40
Ainsworth, Bob 14
Alaska 78
Albarn, Damon 21
Alcoholics Anonymous 26,
  136
Alford, John 27
alkaloids 87-8
Allen, Keith 31
Amazon basin 77
Amendt, Gunter 52
American Society of
  Addiction Medicine 33
amphetamines (speed) 16,
  24, 33-4, 97, 104, 107,
  126, 134
Amsterdam 53, 143
anaesthetic effect of
  cocaine 91, 95, 131

Anderson, Brett 21
Angola 48
anhydrous ethyl ether 109,
  124
Anslinger, Harry 100, 101
Antilles 71
Arbuckle, Fatty 100
Archives of Internal Medicine
  135
Arellano-Felix, Benjamin 60
Arellano-Felix, Ramon
  59-60
Arellano-Felix Organization
  (AFO) 59-60
Argentina 46-7, 55
ASA (Advertising Standards
  Authority) 19-20
Aschenbrandt, Dr Theodore
  90
Asia 45, 48
Atahualpa, Inca 84
AUC (Self-Defence Forces of
  Colombia) 161
Australia 9, 49, 65
Avianca Airlines 106

babies, effects of cocaine on
  135
Bahamas 56
Bank Secrecy Act (US) 150
Bankhead, Tallulah 100
Bankhead, William
  Brockman 100
banknotes
  traces of cocaine on 8
  used for snorting cocaine
    19
Barcelona 97
Barrymore, Michael 27-8

Bashir, Martin 27
Batista, Fulgencio 101
BBC 8, 54, 55, 162, 166
  cocaine use at 29-30
Bear Stearns bank 53
Beatles, The 22
beggars 36-7
Belem (Amazon) 82
Belgium 47
Bells of Hell (New York bar)
  19
Belushi, John 28
Berlin 51-2
Bernal-Madrigal, Alejandro
  168
Bernay, Martha 90
Berne 97
Betancur, Belisario,
  President of Colombia
  108-9, 110
'bingeing' 10, 16, 120
Birmingham 36, 39
Black, Rene 67
Black Market Peso
  Exchange (BMPE) 151,
  153, 154
black people and cocaine
  33-4, 36-7, 95-6, 127, 136,
  168-73
Black Sabbath
  'Snowblind' 21
Blanco, Griselda 105-6
Blériot, Louis 89
Blitz nightclub 23
Blue Hen (yacht) 66
Blues Brothers, The (film) 28
Bogotá 110, 153
Bok, Professor Derek Curtis
  174

Bolivia
   coca production 46, 55,
   56 *bis*, 80, 103, 104
   coca use 83, 85-6
   eradication attempts 93,
   152, 159-60, 163, 164-67
Bonci 121
Bonilla, Lara 108-9, 110
Bonner, Customs
   Commissioner Robert 69
Boston 58
Bowie, David 21
Boyd, Dean 69-70, 152-3,
   154
brain and cocaine (see also
   strokes)118-21
Brazil 46-7, 48, 55, 56, 160
Brigade 2506 (Cuba) 102
Bristol 36, 39, 41
British Crime Survey 8, 40
British Medical Journal
   88-9, 95
Brown, Commander Alan
   32, 34
Brown University,
   Providence 135
Browne, Desmond, QC 24
Brussels 97
Bundestag, cocaine use in 51
Burchill, Julie 27
Bush, President George W
   164
BZ newspaper 51

Cale, JJ 20
Cali 61, 105, 106, 108, 111
Campbell, Naomi 24
Canada 78
Candler, Asa Griggs 93, 95
cannabis (see *marijuana*)
Capone, Al 35-6
Caracol cartel 153
cardiovascular problems
   118, 120, 134
Caribbean 55, 56
Castro, Fidel 102
Catholic Church 86-7, 159
CBS *60 Minutes* programme
   68
Central America, trends in 9
Central Intelligence Agency
   (CIA) 102, 104, 156-8, 164
Chapare region, Bolivia
   164-5

Charles, Prince 25
Charles I of Spain, King 86
Chicago 35-6, 58
children and cocaine 178
   babies 135
Chile 46-7, 78, 81, 101, 103,
   104
Chirrinos, Humberto 162
Christie, Agatha 98
Christison, Sir Robert 88-9
Churches 86-7, 136
CIA (Central Intelligence
   Agency) 102, 104, 156-8,
   164
Cieza de Leon, Pedro 85
Civismo en Marcha party
   107
Clapton, Eric 20
Clash, The
   'I Fought The Law (And
   The Law Won)' 161
Clinton, President Bill 160,
   164, 167
Clovis people 78
clubbing and cocaine 13-17
coca
   anaesthetic properties 76
   crop eradication
   attempts 93, 152, 158,
   159-67, 178
   crop production 55-6, 158
   first users 75-6
   Incas and 78-86
   Spanish Conquistadors
   and 82-7
   species 76-7
   traditional methods of
   consuming 81
   word 'coca' 78
COCA (Conference on Crack
   and Cocaine) 116, 169
Coca-Cola 77, 93, 95
cocaine (see also *addiction*;
   coca; *statistics*)
   costs
      of cocaine 13-14, 37,
      39, 48, 50, 70
      of control
      programmes 167
      of treatment 140, 141,
      146
      distribution
      international traffic
      55-63, 168

methods of smuggling
   63-6
street dealing 38, 41-2
   effects
   anaesthetic 91, 95, 131
   on babies 135
   emotional deadness
   145
   fatigue reduced 89, 125
   guide to side-effects
   131-3
   hunger and thirst
   suspended 89, 125
   paranoia 99
   psychosis 104
   seen as cure for other
   addictions 91-3
   sex improved 30, 103,
   104, 115-18
   strokes 128
   stomach upsets 16
   toxosis ('coke bugs')
   92, 133
   ultimate pleasure 128
   methods of taking
   chewing 9
   drinking 9
   gak blowing (anal
   administration) 22
   injecting (mainlining)
   9, 117
   smoking 9, 10, 123, 126,
   138, 139
   snorting 9, 18, 122, 126
names for 7, 88, 127, 181
purity of 49-50, 57-8
types
   basic paste 57, 94, 123
   crack: qualities 10, 14,
   122-3, 125-27
   crack: social effects
   32-4, 36-41, 70, 138
   freebase 9, 10, 28,
   123-5, 126 *bis*, 138
   powder (cocaine
   hydrochloride) 57-8,
   94, 122, 123-4, 138,
   169
'Cocaine' (song) 20
Cocaine Anonymous World
   Services 130
'Cocaine Lil' (song) 98
cocaine toxosis ('coke
   bugs') 92, 133

Cocolandia laboratories 109
coffee 166
Cohen, Peter and Sas, Arjan
    *Cocaine Use In
    Amsterdam In Non-
    Deviant Subculture* 52-3
Coke-aholics Anonymous
    136-7
Cold War, end of 66
Colombia
    cocaine production 55-6,
    76-7, 158
    cocaine trafficking 55-6,
    58-62, 101, 103-12
    cocaine users 47
    kidnappings 42
    Operation Wire Cutter
    153-4
    Plan Colombia (coca
    reduction) 159, 160-4
Columbus, Christopher 82
Condamine, Charles-Marie
    de la 87
Conference on Crack and
    Cocaine (COCA) 116, 169
Conquistadors 82-7
Contras (see *Nicaragua*)
Cornwall 38-41
costs (see *cocaine [costs]*)
crack (see *cocaine [types]*)
crime (see *street crime;
    violence*)
Cruz, Zenon 165-6
CTR (Currency Transaction
    Reporting) 149, 150
Cuba 101-3, 105
Cyprus 47

Daily Mail 97
    Weekend magazine 25
Daily Telegraph 26, 67, 152
Dallas 58
Darien laboratory 158
DAS (Departamento
    Administrativo de
    Seguridad) 106-7, 153
Daum, Christoph 54
Davis, Johnny 8
DEA (Drug Enforcement
    Administration) 102-3,
    105, 106, 109, 110, 150, 154
    statistics 29, 34, 48, 50,
    70, 150
    website 59, 61

decriminalization of drugs
    177-8
Denmark 47
Denver 58
Departamento Administrativo
    de Seguridad (DAS) 106-7,
    153
Der Spiegel 51-2, 155
Desert News 128
deterrence 179
Devon 39-41
dexedrine 25
Diaz, General Robert 159
Dillehay, Tom 78
distribution (see under
    cocaine)
dogs, sniffer 63
Dominican Republic 56, 58-9
dopamine 117-22 *passim*, 135
Downey, Robert, Jr 140
Doyle, Sir Arthur Conan
    'A Scandal In Bohemia'
    98-9
    'The Final Problem' 99
Dr Don's Coca 93
Dr Tucker's Specific or
    Anglo-American Catarrh
    Powder 93-4
Drug Abuse Warning
    Network 172
Drug Enforcement
    Administration (see *DEA*)

EastEnders (TV) 27
Easy Rider (film) 13, 103
ecstasy (MDMA) 13, 14, 15,
    16, 23, 48, 134, 137
Ecuador 55, 56, 160
Edison, Thomas 90
education, need for 179-80
Edwards, Tracey 67
El Diamante laboratory 109
El Dorado task force 153
El Padrino (Pablo Escobar)
    106-7, 110-12
El Salvador 156
endophilin 118
Ernest Gallo Clinic and
    Research Centre 121
Erythroxylum coca 87
Erythroxylum coca variety
    coca 76
Erythroxylum coca variety
    ipadu 77

*Erythroxylum
    novogranatense* variety
    novogranatense 76-7
*Erythroxylum
    novogranatense* variety
    truxillense 77
Escobar, Pablo 106-7, 110-12,
    155
ether 109, 124
Europe 9, 45, 47-8, 50, 56,
    154, 169
European Union 160

Face magazine 8
Fairbanks, Douglas 100
Faithfull, Marianne 22
FARC (Revolutionary Armed
    Forces of Colombia)
    160-1, 163
fashion modelling and
    cocaine 23-5
FBI (Federal Bureau of
    Investigation) 155
Ferguson, Franklin, Jr 171-2
film industry 99-100
Fleischl-Marxow, Dr Ernst
    von 91
Florida 97, 101-3, 150
Florida University 116
Flynn, Errol 100
Fowler, Robbie 54
Fox, President Vicente 60
France 47
Francisco de Toledo 86
Frankfurt Airport 50-1
Fraser, Robert 22
Freud, Sigmund 75, 78, 90-2
    *The Interpretation Of
    Dreams* 92
Fuentes, Amado Carrillo 61,
    152

Gacha, Jose Gonzalo
    Rodriguez 106
Gallagher, Noel 21 *bis*
Garcilaso de la Vega
    *Royal Commentaries of
    Peru* 83
Gateway Community
    Services, Jacksonville 136
Gatwick Airport 49-50
gay culture 17-18, 34
Geopolitical Drug Watch
    (EU) 51

Germany 47-8, 50-2, 54, 97
 Federal Intelligence
 Service 155
Giesing, Dr Erwin 88
glucose 50
Gold, Dr Mark 131, 133, 134
Gold and Herkov
 'Clinical Aspects Of
 Cocaine And Crack' 138
Goodman, Mike 8
Grateful Dead, The 126
Gray, Aidan 115, 116, 119,
 137-8, 140, 141, 169-70
Groucho Club, London 30-1
Guardian 8, 54, 58, 120, 165
Guatemala 45, 56

Haight-Ashbury Free Clinic
 (HAFC) 33, 104, 126, 136
Haiti 56
Hanna and Hornick
 'Use Of Coca Leaf In
 Southern Peru' 125
Hansard 170
heart problems 118, 120, 134
Heather, Professor Nick 141
Heathrow Airport 49-50,
 68
Heidelberg
 Ophthalmological
 Society 91
Heitt, James 68
Heitt, Laurie 68-9
Hellawell, Keith 54
Helms, Senator Jesse 159
Henao, Herman 66
Henley-on-Thames 68
hepatitis C 117, 138-9
heroin 29, 33, 40, 120, 140
 used with cocaine 28, 40,
 42, 47, 144
Herrera, Helmer ' Pacho' 61,
 105, 111
Het Parool newspaper 71
Hewitt, Superintendent
 Tony 36
High Intensity Drug
 Trafficking Areas (HIDTA)
 conference 69
Hirst, Damien 31
Hitler, Adolf 88
Hitz, Inspector General
 Frederick 157-8
HIV 138, 139-40

HM Customs and Excise
 65-6
Hobbs, Dick 14
Hollywood 99-100
Hoover, J Edgar 155
Hopper, Dennis 26
'Hot Song, The' 98
House of Commons,
 cocaine use at 29
Houston 58
Huancavelica 86
Hu·nuco Valley 80
Huascar, Inca 84
Huayna Capec, Inca 79, 83-4
human rights 165
human sacrifice 79-80
Huppe, Hubert 51
Hutchinson, ASA 154
Huxley, Aldous
 A Treatise On Drugs 177

'I Get A Kick Out Of You'
 (song) 97-8
Ilfracombe 41
Inca people 76, 77-84
'Indian' peoples 125, 143, 167
ING Barings bank 53
Institute of Policy Studies
 (IPS) 149, 162, 164, 171
International Narcotics
 Control Strategy Report
 152
Internet 13, 19, 21
'Irangate' scandal 155-8, 164
Isle of Wight 65-6

Jacobs, Dr Bill 116, 136-7
Jagger, Mick 23
Jamaica/ns 32, 33, 36-6,
 38, 39-41, 49-50, 57, 70
Jaram, Ed 13-14, 15, 32
Jefferson Airplane 126
John, Elton 21
Jones, Ernest
 *The Life And Work Of
 Sigmund Freud* 90
Joplin, Janis 126
*Journal Of Psychoactive
 Drugs* 126
Juarez cartel 60
Jung, George 102
Jurith, Edward 64-5, 66,
 159, 162
Jussieu, Joseph de 87

Kavanagh, Robert 66
Kennedy, President John F
 102
Kerry, John 157
Keystone Studios 100
kidnapping 42-3, 107-8
King, Judge Timothy 66
Kingston Airport 71
Klein, Calvin 24
Koller, Carl 91, 94
Kudlow, Lawrence 53
Kumfort's Cola Extract 93

La Marre, Barbara 100
lactose 50
Lamarck, Jean Chevalier de
 87
Lansky, Meyer 101-2
Lausanne 67
Lavene, Tony 67-8
Le Brun, Didier 66
Leadbelly 98
Ledebur, Kathryn 164-5
Lee, Michael Allen 170
Leeds 36
Lefever, Robin 141
Lehder, Carlos 102, 106
leishmaniasis 85
Liebig's Coca Beef Tonic 93
Liechtenstein 154-5
Liverpool 39
Lockley, Detective Sergeant
 Darren 39-40
London 14, 17, 32, 34-5, 39,
 54, 97
 airports 49-50
 Brixton 37
 Soho 36-7
London Evening Standard
 31
London's Burning (TV) 27
Londono, Jose Santacruz
 105
Los Angeles 58, 171
 Citizens' Commission on
 US Drug Policy 171, 173
Los Angeles Times 125, 157
LSD 16, 126
Lubbock, Stuart 27
Lumière brothers 90

M-19 (Marxist group) 107-8,
 110
McCartney, Sir Paul 22

McKinley, President William 90
McGee, Alan 22
McMahon, Paddy 67
McMahon, Patricia 'Tricia' 67-8, 69
'Maddy' (cocaine user) 17-18
Madrid 97
Mail On Sunday 23
Manchester 39
Manley, Dexter 54-5
Mantegazza, Paolo 88
Mariani, Angelo 89-90
marijuana (cannabis) 16, 27-8, 29, 42
Mass Spec Analytical 8
Maxwell, Robert 155
MDMA (see *ecstasy*)
Meadows rehab clinic, Arizona 26
Medellin 105, 106, 109-12, 158
Merchant, Sarah 129
Merck company 78, 94
methadone 47
methamphetamine 29, 34
Metropolitan Police, London 37, 43, 170
Mexico 55, 56, 59-60, 61, 101, 152
US/Mexican border 58, 62-3
Mexico City 60
Santa Monica Hospital 61
Miami 19, 32-3, 58, 105
Miami Federal Reserve Bank 150
Michael, Michael 58
Middle Market Drug Distribution (UK Home Office study) 14
'Minnie The Moocher' (song) 98
Mirror 24
money laundering 149-55
Monte Verde, Chile 78
Morgan, Piers 24
morphine 91-3
Muerte a Secuestradores (Death to Kidnappers) group 108
mules (carriers) 38, 49-50, 69, 70-72
music and cocaine 13, 19-23, 97-8

Nabokov, Vladimir
'A Matter Of Chance' 98
Nader, Professor Michael 121
Narcotics Anonymous 24
National Crime Squad (NCS) (UK) 65-6
National Drug Control Strategy Report (US) 172
National Institute on Drug Abuse (NIDA) (US) 117, 120, 131, 135, 139
Treating The Brain In Drug Abuse 128
National Security Council (US) 156
Nature magazine 121
NCS (National Crime Squad) (UK) 65-6
Netherlands 47, 50, 56, 70-1
networking 15
neurotransmitters 118-19, 135
NEW-ADAM (New English and Welsh Arrestee Drug Abuse Monitoring) programme 41-2
New Jersey 101
New York 15, 18-19, 33, 58, 59, 107
New York Times 64, 95, 96, 125
New Zealand 49
Newark, US 58
Newsweek 104, 156
Nicaragua 155-58, 164
Niemann, Albert 88, 123
norepinephrine 135
Noriega, Manuel, President of Panama 158-9, 161
Norman, Philip 21
Norman's Cay (Bahamas) 102
Normand, Mabel 100
North, Colonel Oliver 156-7
North America 45, 46
Norway 47
nose, effect of cocaine on 22, 27, 132, 138-9
Nottingham 41-2
Novocain 50
Nueva Granada, Colombia 76

Oasis 23
'What's The Story...' 21
Observer 17, 30, 59, 60, 70, 130

Oceania 45, 49
Ochoa, Jorge 107-8
Ochoa, Marta Nieves 108
Office of Domestic Intelligence (ODI) (US) 58
Office of National Drug Control Policy (ONDCP) (US) 61, 64, 159, 167
older people and cocaine 137
Operation Atrium 36
Operation Eyeful 66
Operation Just Cause 159
Operation Ovidian 36, 39-40
Operation Stirrup 36
Operation Trident 34, 36
Operation Trojan 36
Operation Ventara 36
Operation Wire Cutter 153-4
opiates 169
opium 92-3
oranges 166
Otis, Carre 24-5

Pachacuti, Inca 79
Pachamama (earth goddess) 167
Palmer-Tomkinson, Tara 25-7
Panama 153, 158-9
Paraguay 55
Paris 97
Parke, Davies company 94
Parker, Professor Howard 15
Partnership for a Drug Free America 20
Pastrana, Andres, President of Colombia 161
Pearson, Geoffrey 14
Pearson and Hobbs 41, 42, 43
Pemberton, John 93
Penchef, Laurent 66
Penzance 41
PEPES, Los (People Persecuted by Pablo Escobar) 111
Pistoleros, Los 105-6, 110
Peru (see also *Incas*)
coca leaf consumption 143
cocaine production 46, 55, 56 *bis*, 77, 94, 101, 162
economy 152
eradication programme 93, 159-60

smuggling 68, 103, 104 *bis*
Philadelphia 58
Philip II of Spain 85-6
Phoenix 58
Pinochet, General 104
Pizarro, Francisco 77, 84
plastic surgery 60-1
Plymouth 36, 39-41
poly-drug abuse 47
Porter, Cole 97-8
Portugal 47
Potosì, Bolivia 85-6
President's Click gang 35, 36
Priory rehabilitation centre 170
Promis Recovery Centre, Kent 141
Promises Malibu clinic 140
prostitutes 40, 97, 127
Proust, Marcel 98
Pryor, Richard 28, 124
psychiatric disorders 99, 104, 138
Puerto Asis, Colombia 161
Puerto Rico 56

Quechuan language 78
Quintero, Miguel Caro 60
Quispe, Celestino 166

racial groups and cocaine use 33-4, 36-7, 95-6, 127, 136, 168-73
Ramirez, Jaime 109
Rappe, Virginia 100
Reagan, President Ronald 155, 156, 167
Reevy, Joe 8
rehabilitation 37, 140-1, 170
Reinarman, Professor Craig 'The Social Construction Of Drug Scares' 169 'The Social Impact Of Drugs And The War On Drugs' 167, 168
Release (drugs advice line) 8
Ritz Hotel 31
Rodriguez, Adan Medrano 60
Rodriguez-Orejuela brothers 61, 105, 111
Rolling Stone magazine 103-4

Rolling Stones, The 22
Rome 97
Ross, Ricky 'Freeway Rick' 125
Roxy Music 97
Royal Opera House 31
rubber 87
Rusby, Henry Hurd 94
Russia 66

Safer Clubbing (UK Home Office booklet) 15-16
St Ives 38-9, 40
Salvation Army 144
Samosa, Anastasio 156
San Diego 58
San Francisco 34, 58, 121, 169 Haight-Ashbury district 33
San Jose Mercury News 157
San Ysidro 63
Santa Margarita 82
Santacruz-Londono, Jose 61
Santana, Carlos 126
Savoy Hotel 31
Sayers, Dorothy 98
scapegoating 173-4
Schiphol Airport 70-1
Scotland Yard 32, 34
scouring powder 50
Seattle 58
Select magazine 23
Sennett, Mack 100
11 September attack, effects of 69-71
serotonin 117, 118, 135
Setürner, FWA 87
sex and cocaine use 30, 67, 103, 104, 115-19
sexually transmitted diseases 127
Sheen, Charlie 140
Sherlock Holmes stories 98-9
Shower Posse gang 35
side effects (see *cocaine [effects]*)
Siegel, Benjamin 'Bugsy' 101-2
Siegel, Professor Ron 123-4 *Intoxication* 124
silver mining 85-6
Single Geneva Convention Against Drugs (1962) 93

Sinkinson, Phil 49
Smith, Dr David 33, 104, 126, 136, 146, 168-9
smuggling (see *cocaine [distribution]*)
'smurfing' 150
social class and cocaine use (see also *racial groups*) 7, 36-7, 136-7, 174 professionals and business people 29-32, 52-4, 97 unequal punishments 170-3
Soderbergh, Steven 59
Sonora cartel 60
Sonza, Jose 161
Sorgel, Professor Fritz 51
South Africa 9, 48
South America 9, 45, 46, 160 first users of coca 75-6 Inca people 76, 77, 78-84 prehistory 77-8
Southampton 36
Spaced (Internet club magazine) 13, 32
Spain 33, 47, 48, 50, 55, 56 Conquistadors 82-7
speed (amphetamine) 16, 24, 33-4, 97, 104, 107, 126, 134
'speedballs' (cocaine with heroin/morphine) 28, 92
sport and cocaine 54-5
statistics costs of drug control 167 global use 45 how easy to obtain cocaine 34 males under arrest 29 mortality risk 133 proportion of drug market 40 reduction in coca production 159 smuggling into USA 62, 168 treatment 37 trends in cocaine use 8-9
Stevens, Jodie 141, 142-7, 178
Stewart Marchman Centre, Daytona Beach 136

Strange, Steve 23
Streatfield, Dominic
    *Cocaine: An
    Unauthorized Biography*
    99, 102-3, 168
street crime 32-4, 39-40
street names for cocaine 7,
    181
strokes 128, 133, 134
students 15
studentUK.com 21
Suede
    'We Are The Pigs' 21
Sunday Telegraph 161
Sunday Times 25, 36, 129
    Style magazine 141
Sunderland 41-2
Surinam 71
Svesda Maru (fishing boat)
    65

Take That 22
Tapias, General Fernando
    161
terrorism, war on 69-71,
    163-4
Three Musketeers, The
    (film) 100
Tiffany 31
Tijuana 59
Time Europe magazine 67
Titicaca, Lake 78
Tiwanaku people 78
tobacco 134
Topa, Inca 79
Torres, Frank 109
toxicity 33, 92, 133
Traffic (film) 59
Tranquilandia laboratories
    109
Treaty of Versailles 97
Tree, Sanho 149, 162-4
Trujillo, César Gaviria 111
Trujillo coca 77
turf wars 34-5, 40-1, 42
Turkey 47
Tyrrell, Michael 65-6

Ungless, Dr Mark 121
United Kingdom 36-42, 47,
    49, 50, 70, 170-1

HM Customs and Excise
    65-6
Home Office publications
    13, 15, 14
National Crime Squad
    (NCS) 65-6
United Nations
    Commission of Enquiry on
    the Coca Leaf (1949) 101
    GIDT (*Global Illicit Drug
    Trends*) report 9, 45, 46,
    48, 49, 56
    special conference on
    drugs (1998) 55
    UNDCP (UN Drug Control
    Programme) 45, 46, 76,
    158, 162
    UNODCCP (UN Office of
    Drug Control and Crime
    Prevention) 47-8, 49, 50
United States of America
    18-19
    Coast Guards 64
    Customs Service 62, 149,
    151, 154
    Department of Justice
    quoted 12
    early use of cocaine
    92-3, 96-7
    hospital admissions 50
    'Irangate' scandal
    155-58, 164
    money laundering
    149-52
    price of cocaine 48, 50
    proportion of cocaine
    users 9
    quantities of cocaine
    seized 56
    system of dealing 42
University of California 121,
    123, 139, 173
University of Florida 116, 131,
    133
University of Gottingen
    123
University of Northumbria
    141
University of Texas 118
Ure, Midge 23
Uruguay 55

USCS (United States
    Customs Service) 62,
    149, 151, 154
Vandenberghe, Patricio 162
Vasquez, Jorge Luis Ochoa
    106
Venezuela 55, 56, 153, 160
Verne, Jules 89
Vespucci, Amerigo 82
Viagra 117-18
Vietnam War 173
Villanueva, Mario 60
Vin Mariani 89-90
Viracocha, Inca 78-9
Visage
    'Fade To Grey' 23
VH1 (TV channel) 19-20
violence 14, 32-3, 34-5, 42-3,
    60, 95, 106, 107, 110-11
Volkow, Dr Nora 118, 120
Vyner, Harriet
    Groovy Bob 22

Wake Forest University 121
'war on drugs' 112, 179
'war on terror' 69-70,
    163-4
Washton, Dr Arnold 53-4
Webb, Gary 157
Wells, HG 90
Westbrook, Danniella 27
Williams, Superintendent
    Carl 36
Williams, Robbie 22-3
Wilson, Martin 67
wired.com (Internet
    magazine) 17
Wöhler, Friedrich 87-8
Wood, Ronnie 22
Wright, Superintendent
    Gladstone 70, 95

Yale University 135
Yardie gangs 32, 35-6
Young, Toby 30-1
    On The Way To Work 31
Yungas, Bolivia 80, 166-7

Zedillo, Ernesto, President
    of Mexico 152
zero tolerance 13

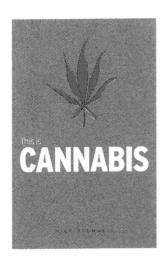

In the 4,700 years since its first recorded use, cannabis has been respected as a highly useful source of fibre, food, and medicine and vilified as a social menace. Society in the 21st century seems to be of both opinions: doctors and scientists spend millions exploiting its medicinal value and thousands of people travel to Amsterdam each weekend to sit in cafés to smoke copious amounts of dope free from molestation, yet taking less than 30g (1oz) back into their own countries is an offence and public figures who admit to smoking cannabis in their youth claim that they did so without inhaling.

This Is Cannabis does not preach the benefits or the deficits of cannabis; instead, it aims to provide the facts about cannabis in an authoritative, straightforward way, outlining the history, laws, and culture that have accreted around it, its effects on health, and the booming commercial potential.

ISBN 1 86074 399 4

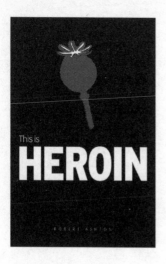

This is
HEROIN

ROBERT ASHTON

Heroin was a terrible mistake. Its creator, English researcher CR Alder Wright, was seeking a non-addictive alternative to morphine, already a social problem. He failed. While morphine is up to 1,000 per cent stronger than opium, heroin is eight times more potent than morphine and just as addictive.

In the UK alone, annual consumption of pure heroin is between 28,000kg and 36,000kg (25 and 32 tons) and just one kilo (2¼lb) distributed at street level can result in 220 victims of burglary and £220,000 [$320,000] worth of theft. In the USA, 87 per cent of the drug's 2.4 million users are aged under 26, while the average age of experimentation has fallen to only 15.

Heroin can mean death for the user by overdose, poison, or murder, as well as infection of AIDS and hepatitis from dirty needles. But what are the direct physical effects? How addictive is the drug? What are the stages of withdrawal? Can you use and come off safely? Would a legalized, controlled and regulated supply of heroin reduce overdose deaths and enable users to live higher-quality lives? International in its scope and unshrinkingly frank, *This Is Heroin* presents the social and physical reality of the world's most demonized drug.

ISBN 1 86074 424 9

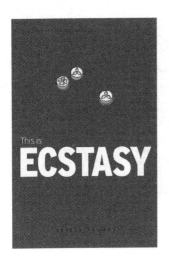

Ecstasy is a problem child. One of the most notorious designer drugs to have risen out of the '80s rave scene, a young drug embraced by the young, the stuff of peer pressure rather than caution. An official survey estimates that in the UK 430,000 users spend a total of £300 million ($441 million) a year on ecstasy, taking between one and five pills a night, while unofficial sources have it that consumption is twice this figure. To date, there have been around 90 E-related deaths reported in the UK and around 40 in the United States, where E is no longer just a club drug but is increasingly available in schools and homes, finding new customers in ex-cocaine users.

This Is Ecstasy presents the very latest information from around the world concerning the drug's culture, manufacture, and trafficking, its medical origin (it was once nicknamed 'penicillin for the soul'), its short- and long-term effects on health, the legal and political ramifications of its use, and the consequent backlash from supporters of the drug.

In the words of Alexander Shulgin, the remarkable scientist who nurtured ecstasy through its infancy, 'Be informed, then choose.'

ISBN 1 86074 426 5

Also available
in this series

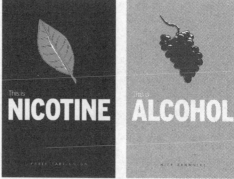